Physical Medicine and Rehabilitation: Principles and Practice

Physical Medicine and Rehabilitation: Principles and Practice

Patricia Jackson

MURPHY & MOORE
www.murphy-moorepublishing.com

Published by Murphy & Moore Publishing,
1 Rockefeller Plaza,
New York City, NY 10020, USA
www.murphy-moorepublishing.com

Physical Medicine and Rehabilitation: Principles and Practice
Patricia Jackson

International Standard Book Number: 978-1-63987-428-6 (Hardback)

Cataloging-in-Publication Data

Physical medicine and rehabilitation : principles and practice / Patricia Jackson.
p. cm.
Includes bibliographical references and index.
ISBN 978-1-63987-428-6
1. Medicine, Physical. 2. Medical rehabilitation. I. Jackson, Patricia.
RM700 .P49 2022
615.82--dc23

TABLE OF CONTENTS

PREFACE

This book aims to help a broader range of students by exploring a wide variety of significant topics related to this discipline. It will help students in achieving a higher level of understanding of the subject and excel in their respective fields. This book would not have been possible without the unwavered support of my senior professors who took out the time to provide me feedback and help me with the process. I would also like to thank my family for their patience and support.

Physical medicine and rehabilitation is the sub-field of medicine that deals with the enhancement and restoration of functional ability and quality of life of those with physical disabilities and impairments. It is also known as physiatrics and physiatry. This field deals with restoring optimal functioning of injured muscles, ligaments, bones or nervous system. It is used to treat spinal cord injuries, amputation, traumatic brain and other debilitating injuries. The field is majorly concerned with the functioning of disabled part of the body for which there is no known cure. It uses the process of goal setting to treat a person undergoing rehabilitation for an acquired impairment. Some of the subspecialties within this field are pain medicine, sports medicine, neuromuscular medicine, pediatric rehabilitation medicine, and hospice and palliative medicine. This book provides comprehensive insights into the field of physical medicine and rehabilitation. It is an upcoming field of medicine that has undergone rapid development over the past few decades. This book is a complete source of knowledge on the present status of this important field.

A brief overview of the book contents is provided below:

Chapter - Introduction

The branch of medicine that deals with the enhancement and restoration of functional abilities and quality of life for people with disabilities is referred to as physical medicine and rehabilitation. It treats patients suffering from spinal cord injuries, brain injuries, amputation, etc. This is an introductory chapter which will briefly introduce about physical medicine and rehabilitation.

Chapter - Specializations in Physical Medicine

There are various sub-specializations that fall under the domain of physical medicine such as sports medicine, neuromuscular medicine, hospice and palliative medicine, etc. This chapter closely examines these sub-specializations of physical medicine to provide an extensive understanding of the subject.

Chapter - Sports Injuries and their Treatment

Sports injuries can occur due to overtraining, lack of conditioning, improper form and technique, etc. Some common injuries are shin splints, tennis elbow, Achilles tendon rupture, rotator cuff tendinitis, lumbar spine pain, etc. The topics elaborated in this chapter will help in gaining a better perspective of the sports injuries and treatment.

Chapter – Physical Therapies

Physical therapies treat the deformities and some injuries by using different physical methods and specially designed exercises. It includes cryotherapy, dry needling, hydrotherapy, diathermy, electrotherapy, heat therapy, soft tissue therapy, etc. This chapter sheds light on the various physical therapies for a thorough understanding of the subject.

Chapter – Rehabilitation Exercises

Rehabilitation exercises help in restoring lost skills and regaining maximum self-sufficiency. Stretching exercises, foam roller exercises, plyometric exercises, etc. are a few rehabilitation exercises. This chapter has been carefully written to provide an extensive understanding of these rehabilitation exercises.

Patricia Jackson

Introduction

1

- **Physical Medicine and Rehabilitation**
- **Physical Therapy Attack**
- **Rehabilitation**

The branch of medicine that deals with the enhancement and restoration of functional abilities and quality of life for people with disabilities is referred to as physical medicine and rehabilitation. It treats patients suffering from spinal cord injuries, brain injuries, amputation, etc. This is an introductory chapter which will briefly introduce about physical medicine and rehabilitation.

Physical Medicine and Rehabilitation

Physical medicine and rehabilitation, also called physiatry or rehabilitation medicine is a medical specialty concerned with the diagnosis, treatment, and prevention of physical impairments, particularly those associated with disorders of the muscles, nerves, bones, or brain. This specialized medical service is generally aimed at rehabilitating persons disabled by pain or ailments affecting the motor functions of the body. Physical medicine is one means employed to assist these patients to return to a comfortable and productive life, often despite the persistence of a medical problem.

For centuries people have used such natural physical agents as hot springs and sunlight to treat ailments, but the development of physical medicine as a specialized medical service took place largely after World War I. Two factors influenced its growth in the 20th century—epidemic poliomyelitis and the two World Wars—both of which created large numbers of seriously handicapped young people. Physical medicine was definitively established through the American physician Howard A. Rusk's efforts to rehabilitate wounded soldiers during and after World War II. Physical medicine then became available for the treatment of patients with such diverse problems as fractures, burns, tuberculosis, painful backs, strokes, nerve and spinal cord injuries, diabetes, birth defects, arthritis, and vision and speech impairments. Physical medicine is closely associated with orthopedic surgery, but it is prescribed by physicians and surgeons in all branches of medicine. Physicians who specialize in physical medicine are called physiatrists.

The objectives of physical medicine are relief of pain, improvement or maintenance of functions such as strength and mobility, training in the most effective method of performing essential activities, and testing of function in various areas. Tests cover such fields as muscle strength, degree of joint mobility, breathing capacity, and muscular coordination.

The therapeutic means most commonly employed include heat, massage, exercise, electrical currents, and functional training. Since the 1970s these basic means have been supplemented and enhanced by psychological counseling, occupational therapy, and a variety of other treatments which may be used in concert to help the disabled person achieve the fullest possible life despite the persistence of medical problems.

Heat is used generally to stimulate circulation and to relieve pain in the area treated. For example, in diathermy heat may be applied by shortwave or microwave radiation or by ultrasound. Other forms of heat therapy include the use of hot, moist compresses and hydrotherapy (immersion in hot water). Massage primarily aids circulation and relieves local pain or muscle spasm.

Exercise, the most varied and widely used of all physical treatments, is usually designed to do one or more of three things: increase the amount of motion in a joint, increase the strength in a muscle, or train a muscle to contract and relax in useful coordination with other muscles. In addition to its obvious use following stiffness or paralysis, exercise may be used to improve the breathing of patients with lung disorders, assist circulation, relax tense muscles, and correct faulty posture.

In the late 20th century high technology was increasingly harnessed in efforts to rehabilitate paraplegics, quadriplegics, and others with severely impaired motor functions. Microcomputers were developed that could send precisely coordinated jolts of electricity directly into the muscles of such patients, mimicking the cerebral impulses that could no longer reach their muscle destinations because of a severed spinal cord. The microcomputers' sophisticated programs enable them to contract a patient's muscles in unison so that he can actually stand and sit, walk, and even use his hands to perform relatively fine movements. Such devices were still in the experimental stage and were costly to make and use, but they seemed to be the most promising development yet in efforts to restore the power of movement to nerve injury victims.

Other, less ambitious devices to help paralyzed patients include wheelchairs with specially equipped control systems that can be operated by the mouth and teeth movements of a quadriplegic. Mobile robotic arms have been developed that are equipped with a video camera so that they can move safely and intelligently about a patient's house. These personal robots can receive and execute oral commands from the patient to perform such simple household tasks as filling a glass with water or taking a book off a shelf.

Functional training teaches the impaired individual how to carry out most safely and effectively the activities of daily life. This training may mean learning to use crutches, a brace, or an artificial arm; or it may involve working out and practicing the movements required to do housework with the use of only one hand or the way to board public transportation with a stiff leg. Such training often requires long hours of practice; it may be facilitated by use of devices that make it easier to fasten buttons, hold a fork, or dial a telephone.

Physical medicine and rehabilitation underwent a rapid expansion during the late 20th century, largely because of the development of antibiotics and other fundamental advances in modern medicine, which not only save the lives of many who would not have survived illness or injury in earlier decades but also prolong life in general.

Physical medicine and rehabilitation are carried out by a "rehabilitation team," headed by a physiatrist who coordinates the team's efforts and assesses the areas of functioning in which the patient can improve. The physical therapist uses exercise to improve the patient's muscle strength and functioning, and a rehabilitation engineer may provide a special mechanical aid or device to assist that functioning. Meanwhile a rehabilitation nurse keeps track of the patient's physical condition and provides him with basic medical care, while a psychological counselor helps the patient cope with the discouragement or depression produced by the condition of physical disability. Respiratory or speech therapists may also be brought in to assist the patient with breathing or speaking difficulties. Eventually an occupational therapist and a social worker will help the patient adjust to life outside of the rehabilitation institute.

Types of Physical Medicine and Rehabilitation

Various injuries and illnesses can cause damage to the body and impede movement, cause pain, or generally reduce your physical health. Physical medicine is the branch of medicine that focuses on rehabilitation, using a variety of medical and therapeutic procedures to restore your body to healthy condition. Although physical medicine centers tend to be interdisciplinary, the specialists at these centers are usually trained in certain types of physical medicine and rehabilitation. The following are some of the most common types of injuries and health conditions that prevent people from living vital, active, and healthy lives.

Bone Health

One of the most popular branches of physical medicine is bone health. Bone specialists are experts in human skeletal structure and anatomy. They study the various ways in which injuries or disorders of the bones affect the rehabilitation and recovery process. One of the most common causes of bone health issues is an improperly healed fracture. With smaller hairline fractures, it is possible not to even know that a bone was ever broken. When bones are fractured, they almost always need to be reset and placed in a cast to prevent movement. Setting a bone ensures that it will heal properly and quickly. When a bone is improperly set or allowed to heal without setting at all, you will most likely need physical therapy to correct the damage. In some cases, physical therapy specialists will break an improperly healed bone again in order to reset the recovery process properly. Bone specialists frequently practice rehabilitation with victims of car accidents and sports injuries.

Joint Health

Joint health is another popular subfield of physical medicine. Whether you have joint issues as the result of an injury, long-term wear, or an arthritic condition, joint specialists can help you improve mobility and lessen the pain you experience. Physical therapists generally take a holistic approach to joint health. Your joint health specialist will likely ask you a variety of questions about your daily activities before starting you on a rehabilitation and recovery plan. Regular mild exercise is essential to joint recovery and rehabilitation, so the rehabilitation process will almost always begin with physical therapy. Physical medicine may involve the addition of pharmacological treatment as well as the exercises and stretches used in physical therapy, creating a comprehensive rehabilitation plan designed for maximum recovery.

Nerve Injuries

Nerve injuries are generally caused by physical trauma, but they may also be due to neurological conditions. Recovery and rehabilitation from nerve injuries is often difficult, and nerve health remains one of the most widely used forms of physical medicine. The nervous system is a complex part of the body, capable of sending impulses that make it feel as if a missing body part is still in pain or even triggering severe pain without any apparent cause. The recovery process can be aided by nerve specialists who understand the complex structure of the nervous system. Your physical medicine specialist will tailor a plan to meet your needs, whether your nerve problems are the result of an injury or another medical condition. This is one of the most exciting frontiers because neuroscientists are constantly making new discoveries that physical medicine specialists can use in treatment.

Pain Therapy

Pain therapy is a new and exciting branch of physical medicine that opens doors of recovery to patients with various pain disorders and injuries that were previously thought untreatable. The process of recovery and rehabilitation from a pain disorder can be long and difficult, but with help from the right physical medicine professionals, it is not impossible. Physical rehabilitation and recovery is a holistic branch of medicine that gives patients access to specialists in a variety of fields. Pain therapy is an interdisciplinary subfield of physical medicine, attracting knowledgeable specialists from all the branches of physical medicine that deal with pain. Through a blend of pharmacological treatment options, physical therapy, and lifestyle changes, physical specialists have seen encouraging results in the rehabilitation and recovery of their patients with chronic pain. Some physical medicine practitioners even use methods that can completely eliminate chronic pain, depending on the individual.

Sports Injuries

Sports injuries are one of the most common reasons for seeking treatment at a physical medicine center. Many people don't take rehabilitation and recovery from sports injuries as seriously as they should. Athletes often shun rehabilitation treatment and prolong the recovery process unnecessarily by continuing to play while injured. Straining the joints, ligaments, muscles, and bones hinders recovery and makes rehabilitation even more difficult. To allow for proper rehabilitation and recovery, athletes must give their bodies a chance to heal from their injuries with adequate rest and physical therapy. Because the recovery and rehabilitation process can be so difficult for athletes, many choose to go through recovery in a physical medicine inpatient center vs. outpatient rehab because they can be regularly monitored. Recovery takes time, but checking into a physical medicine center can actually speed the rehabilitation process, because it forces injured people to take the time they need for recovery.

Congenital Conditions

In addition to medical problems that occur due to specific injuries, physical medicine also deals with congenital problems, or those that affect an individual from birth. Various diseases and disorders can affect the way your body works, causing distressing symptoms that limit your range of motion and inhibit your quality of life. Physical therapy is an ideal way to treat the movement issues that can be caused by congenital health conditions. Although many of these conditions are incurable, physical medicine provides numerous options for rehabilitation and recovery. It is possible to be in recovery from some of the more troubling symptoms of congenital illnesses through the help of a reliable physical medicine specialist.

Brain Disorders

Brain disorders are another common part of the physical medicine spectrum. Brain disorders often occur as the result of head trauma, tumors, surgery, or other forms of physical injury. Unlike psychological problems, brain disorders have a physical cause, so physical rehabilitation and recovery is almost always possible. The recovery and rehabilitation process involves working with a physical specialist who understands the various brain disorders and their causes. Recovery times vary depending on the severity of the disorder and the extent of the damage done to the brain. The brain is a sensitive organ, so rehabilitation for brain disorders is often more complex than rehabilitation in other areas of physical medicine. Physical specialists may work with other professionals to facilitate the recovery process and manage all symptoms, both physical and psychological.

General Physical Medicine

While some physical rehabilitation and recovery practitioners choose to specialize in one of the specific types of physical medicine and rehabilitation, others choose to become general practitioners of physical medicine. Physical rehabilitation and recovery is a diverse area of study, and general physical medicine practitioners see patients with a variety of issues, helping them with the rehabilitation process. Recovery is possible even if your issues stem from several different parts of the physical medicine spectrum. Finding the best rehabilitation treatment center or physical medicine rehabilitation program can be an important first step in your journey to recovery.

Physical Therapy

In physical therapy, trained professionals evaluate and treat abnormal physical function related to, for example, an injury, disability, disease or condition.

A physical therapist is a trained and licensed medical professional with experience in diagnosing physical abnormalities, restoring physical function and mobility, maintaining physical function, and promoting physical activity and proper function.

Licensed physical therapists can be found in a range of healthcare settings including outpatient offices, private practices, hospitals, rehab centers, nursing homes, home health, sports and fitness settings, schools, hospices, occupational settings, government agencies, and research centers.

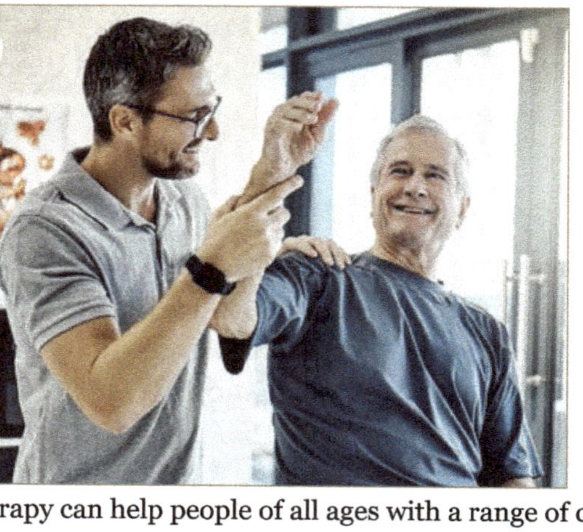

Physical therapy can help people of all ages with a range of conditions.

A physical therapist helps take care of patients in all phases of healing, from initial diagnosis through the restorative and preventive stages of recovery. Physical therapy may be a standalone option, or it may support other treatments.

Some patients are referred to a physical therapist by their doctor, but other seek therapy themselves.

Whichever way a patient come to a physical therapist, they can expect to:

- Undergo a physical exam and evaluation, including a health history and certain testing procedures, including evaluation of posture, movement and flexibility, and of muscle and joint motion and performance.
- Receive a clinical diagnosis, prognosis, plan of care and short and long term goals.
- Receive physical therapy treatment and intervention based on the therapist's evaluation and diagnosis.
- Receive self-management recommendations.

Patients often train with a physical therapist in exercises that they can do at home, to help them function more effectively.

Common Conditions

Physical therapists can treat a wide variety of medical conditions, depending on their specialty.

Some conditions that can benefit from this type of treatment are:

- Cardiopulmonary conditions, such as chronic obstructive pulmonary disease (COPD), cystic fibrosis (CF) and post-myocardial infarction (MI).
- Hand therapy for conditions such as carpal tunnel syndrome and trigger finger.
- Musculoskeletal dysfunction such as back pain, rotator cuff tears, and temporomandibular joint disorders (TMJ).
- Neurological conditions such as stroke, spinal cord injuries, Parkinson's disease, multiple sclerosis, vestibular dysfunction, and traumatic brain injuries.
- Pediatric conditions such as developmental delays, cerebral palsy, and muscular dystrophy.
- Sports-related injuries, such as concussion and tennis elbow.
- Women's health and pelvic floor dysfunction, such as urinary incontinence and lymphedema.

Other cases that may benefit include burns, wound care, and diabetic ulcers.

Benefits of Physical Therapy

Depending on the reason for treatment, the benefits of physical therapy include:

- Pain management with reduced need for opioids.
- Avoiding surgery.
- Improved mobility and movement.
- Recovery from injury or trauma.
- Recovery from stroke or paralysis.
- Fall prevention.
- Improved balance.
- Management of age-related medical problems.

A sports therapist can help an athlete to maximize their performance through strengthening specific parts of the body and using muscles in new ways.

A healthcare provider or physical therapist can advise individuals about the benefits specific to their personal medical history and their need for treatment.

Types

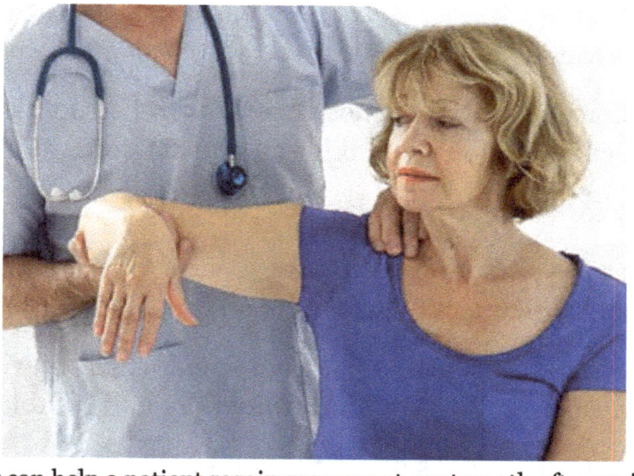

Physical therapy can help a patient regain movement or strength after an injury or illness.

As with any medical practice, a variety of therapies can be applied to treat a range of conditions.

- Orthopedic physical therapy: Treats musculoskeletal injuries, involving the muscles, bones, ligaments, fascias, and tendons. It is suitable for medical conditions such as fractures, sprains, tendonitis, bursitis, chronic medical problems, and rehabilitation or recovery from orthopedic surgery. Patients may undergo treatment with joint mobilizations, manual therapy, strength training, mobility training, and other modalities.

- Geriatric physical therapy: It can help older patients who develop conditions that affect their mobility and physical function, including arthritis, osteoporosis, Alzheimer's disease, hip and joint replacement, balance disorders, and incontinence. This type of intervention aims to restore mobility, reduce pain and increase physical fitness levels.
- Neurological physical therapy: It can help people with neurological disorders and conditions such as Alzheimer's disease, brain injury, cerebral palsy, multiple sclerosis, Parkinson's disease, spinal cord injury, and stroke. Treatment may aim to increase limb responsiveness, treat paralysis, and reverse increase muscles strength by reducing muscle atrophy.
- Cardiovascular and pulmonary rehabilitation: It can benefit people affected by some cardiopulmonary conditions and surgical procedures. Treatment can increase physical endurance and stamina.
- Pediatric physical therapy: Aims to diagnose, treat, and manage conditions that affect infants, children, and adolescents, including developmental delays, cerebral palsy, spina bifida, torticollis and other conditions that impact the musculoskeletal system.
- Wound care therapy: It can help to ensure that a healing wound is receiving adequate oxygen and blood by way of improved circulation. Physical therapy may include the use of manual therapies, electric stimulation, compression therapy and wound care.
- Vestibular therapy: Aims to treat balance problems that can result from inner ear conditions. Vestibular physical therapy involves a number of exercises and manual techniques that can help patients regain their normal balance and coordination.
- Decongestive therapy: It can help to drain accumulated fluid in patients with lymphedema and other conditions that involve fluid accumulation.
- Pelvic floor rehabilitation: It can help treat urinary or fecal incontinence, urinary urgency and pelvic pain in men and women as a result of injuries or surgery, or because of certain conditions.

Apart from physical manipulation, physical therapy treatment may involve:

- Ultrasound, to promote blood flow and healing by heating the tendons, muscles, and tissues.

- Phonophoresis, which uses ultrasound to deliver certain medications such as topical steroids. This can decrease the presence of inflammation.
- Electrical stimulation, or E-stim, which uses topical electrodes on the skin to reduce pain and increase functional capabilities. One type of E-stim is transcutaneous electrical nerve stimulation (TENS). At times, anti-inflammatory medications are used with certain E-stim modalities and is referred to as iontophoresis.
- Heat, moist heat and cold therapy.
- Light therapy, in which special lights and lasers are used to treat certain medical conditions.

The physical therapist will recommend the most appropriate treatment.

Rehabilitation

Rehabilitation is care that can help you get back, keep, or improve abilities that you need for daily life. These abilities may be physical, mental, and/or cognitive (thinking and learning). You may have lost them because of a disease or injury, or as a side effect from a medical treatment. Rehabilitation can improve your daily life and functioning.

Need of Rehabilitation

Rehabilitation is for people who have lost abilities that they need for daily life. Some of the most common causes include

- Injuries and trauma, including burns, fractures (broken bones), traumatic brain injury, and spinal cord injuries.
- Stroke.
- Severe infections.
- Major surgery.
- Side effects from medical treatments, such as from cancer treatments.
- Certain birth defects and genetic disorders.
- Developmental disabilities.
- Chronic pain, including back and neck pain.

Goals of Rehabilitation

The overall goal of rehabilitation is to help you get your abilities back and regain independence. But the specific goals are different for each person. They depend on what caused the problem, whether the cause is ongoing or temporary, which abilities you lost, and how severe the problem is. For example:

- A person who has had a stroke may need rehabilitation to be able to dress or bathe without help.
- An active person who has had a heart attack may go through cardiac rehabilitation to try to return to exercising.
- Someone with a lung disease may get pulmonary rehabilitation to be able to breathe better and improve their quality of life.

Rehabilitation Program

When you get rehabilitation, you often have a team of different health care providers helping you. They will work with you to figure out your needs, goals, and treatment plan. The types of treatments that may be in a treatment plan include:

- Assistive devices, which are tools, equipment, and products that help people with disabilities move and function.
- Cognitive rehabilitation therapy to help you relearn or improve skills such as thinking, learning, memory, planning, and decision making.
- Mental health counseling.
- Music or art therapy to help you express your feelings, improve your thinking, and develop social connections.
- Nutritional counseling.
- Occupational therapy to help you with your daily activities.
- Physical therapy to help your strength, mobility, and fitness.
- Recreational therapy to improve your emotional well-being through arts and crafts, games, relaxation training, and animal-assisted therapy.
- Speech-language therapy to help with speaking, understanding, reading, writing and swallowing.
- Treatment for pain.
- Vocational rehabilitation to help you build skills for going to school or working at a job.

Depending on your needs, you may have rehabilitation in the providers' offices, a hospital, or an inpatient rehabilitation center. In some cases, a provider may come to your home. If you get care in your home, you will need to have family members or friends who can come and help with your rehabilitation.

Rehabilitation in Sport

Rehabilitation is the restoration of optimal form (anatomy) and function (physiology).

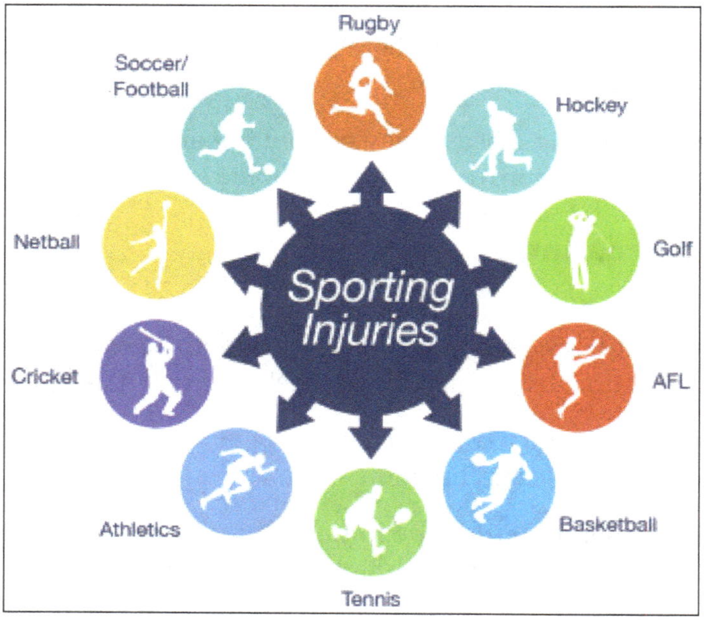

It is a process designed to minimize the loss associated with acute injury or chronic disease, to promote recovery, and to maximize functional capacity, fitness and performance.

Musculoskeletal injuries are an inevitable result of sport participation. Football has the highest incidence of catastrophic injuries, with gymnastics and ice hockey close behind. Tissue injury from sports can be classified as macrotraumatic and microtraumatic.

- Macrotraumatic injuries are usually due to a strong force – such as a fall, accident, collision or laceration – and are more common in contact sports such as football and rugby. These injuries can be primary (due to direct tissue damage) or secondary (due to transmission of forces or release of inflammatory mediators and other cytokinesis).
- Microtraumatic injuries are chronic injuries that result from overuse of a structure such as a muscle, joint, ligament, or tendon. This type of injury is more common in sports such as swimming, cycling and rowing.

The process of rehabilitation should start as early as possible after an injury and form a continuum with other therapeutic interventions. It can also start before or immediately after surgery when an injury requires a surgical intervention.

Rehabilitation Plan

The rehabilitation plan must take into account the fact that the objective of the patient (the athlete) is to return to the same activity and environment in which the injury occurred. Functional capacity after rehabilitation should be the same, if not better, than before injury.

The ultimate goal of the rehabilitation process is to limit the extent of the injury, reduce or reverse the impairment and functional loss, and prevent, correct or eliminate altogether the disability.

Multidisciplinary Approach

The rehabilitation of the injured athlete is managed by a multidisciplinary team with a physician functioning as the leader and coordinator of care. The team includes, but is not limited to, sports physicians, physiatrists (rehabilitation medicine practitioners), orthopaedists, physiotherapists, rehabilitation workers, physical educators, coaches, athletic trainers, psychologists, and nutritionists. The rehabilitation team works closely with the athlete and the coach to establish the rehabilitation goals, to discuss the progress resulting from the various interventions, and to establish the time frame for the return of the athletes to training and competition.

Communication is a vital factor. A lack of communication between medical providers, strength and conditioning specialists, and team coaches can slow or prevent athletes from returning to peak capability and increase the risk of new injuries and even more devastating reinjuries.

Principles

Principles are the foundation upon which rehabilitation is based. Here are seven principles of rehabilitation, which can be remembered by the mnemonic: ATC IS IT.

- A: Avoid aggravation. It is important not to aggravate the injury during the rehabilitation process. Therapeutic exercise, if administered incorrectly or without good judgment, has the potential to exacerbate the injury, that is, make it worse.
- T: Timing. The therapeutic exercise portion of the rehabilitation program should begin as soon as possible—that is, as soon as it can occur without causing aggravation. The sooner patients can begin the exercise portion of the rehabilitation program, the sooner they can return to full activity. Following injury, rest is sometimes necessary, but too much rest can actually be detrimental to recovery.

- C: Compliance. Without a compliant patient, the rehabilitation program will not be successful. To ensure compliance, it is important to inform the patient of the content of the program and the expected course of rehabilitation.
- I: Individualization. Each person responds differently to an injury and to the subsequent rehabilitation program. Even though an injury may seem the same in type and severity as another, undetectable differences can change an individual's response to it. Individual physiological and chemical differences profoundly affect a patient's specific responses to an injury.
- S: Specific sequencing. A therapeutic exercise program should follow a specific sequence of events. This specific sequence is determined by the body's physiological healing response.
- I: Intensity. The intensity level of the therapeutic exercise program must challenge the patient and the injured area but at the same time must not cause aggravation. Knowing when to increase intensity without overtaxing the injury requires observation of the patient's response and consideration of the healing process.
- T: Total patient. It must be considered the total patient in the rehabilitation process. It is important for the unaffected areas of the body to stay finely tuned. This means keeping the cardiovascular system at a preinjury level and maintaining range of motion, strength, coordination, and muscle endurance of the uninjured limbs and joints. The whole body must be the focus of the rehabilitation program, not just the injured area. Providing the patient with a program to keep the uninvolved areas in peak condition, rather than just rehabilitating the injured area, will help to better prepare the patient physically and psychologically for when the injured area is completely rehabilitated.

Components

Regardless of the specifics of the injury, however, here are fundamental components that need to be included in all successful rehabilitation programs:

Pain Management

Medications are a mainstay of treatment in the injured athlete - both for their pain relief and healing properties. It is recommended that they need to be used judiciously with a distinct regard for the risks and side effects as well as the potential benefits, which include pain relief and early return to play. Therapeutic modalities play a small, but important, part in the rehabilitation of sports injuries. They may help to decrease pain and edema to allow an exercise-based rehabilitation programme to proceed. By understanding the physiological basis of these modalities, a safe and appropriate treatment choice can be made, but its effectiveness will ultimately depend upon the patient's individualized and subjective response to treatment.

Flexibility and Joint ROM

Injury or surgery can result in decreased joint ROM mainly due to fibrosis and wound contraction. Besides that, it is common for post-injury flexibility to be diminished as a result of muscle spasm, inflammation, swelling and pain. In addition to impacting the injured area, this also affects the joints above and below the problem, and creates motor pattern issues. Flexibility training is an important component of rehabilitation in order to minimize the decrease in joint ROM. Also, a variety of stretching techniques can be used in improving range of motion, including PNF, ballistic stretching and static stretching.

Strength and Endurance

Injuries to the musculoskeletal system could result in skeletal muscle hypotrophy and weakness, loss of aerobic capacity and fatigability. During rehabilitation after a sports injury it is important to try to maintain cardiovascular endurance. Thus regular bicycling, one-legged bicycling or arm cycling, an exercise programme in a pool using a wet vest or general major muscle exercise programmes with relatively high intensity and short rest periods (circuit weight training) can be of major importance.

Proprioception and Coordination

Proprioception can be defined as 'a special type of sensitivity that informs about the sensations of the deep organs and of the relationship between muscles and joints'. Loss of proprioception occurs with injury to ligaments, tendons, or joints, and also with immobilization. Proprioceptive re-education has to get the muscular receptors working, in order to provide a rapid motor response. Restoration of proprioception is an important part of rehabilitation. The treatment has to be adapted to each individual, considering the type of injury and the stress to which the athlete will be exposed when practicing his or her sport.

Coordination can be defined as 'the capacity to perform movements in a smooth, precise and controlled manner'. Rehabilitation techniques increasingly refer to neuromuscular re-education. Improving coordination depends on repeating the positions and movements associated with different sports and correct training. It has to begin with simple activities, performed slowly and perfectly executed, gradually increasing in speed and complexity. The technician should make sure that the athlete performs these movements unconsciously, until they finally become automatic.

Functional Rehabilitation

All rehabilitation programs must take into account, and reproduce, the activities and movements required when the athlete returns to the field post-injury. The goal of function-based rehabilitation programmes is the return of the athlete to optimum athletic function. Optimal athletic function is the result of physiological motor activations creating specific biomechanical motions and positions using intact anatomical structures to generate forces and actions.

The use of Orthotics

The use of orthotic devices to support musculoskeletal function and the correction of muscle imbalances and inflexibility in uninjured areas should receive the attention of the rehabilitation team. Appropriate orthotic application will result in restraint forces that oppose an undesired motion. A complete orthotic prescription should include the patient's diagnosis, consider the type of footwear to be used, include the joints it encompasses and specify the desired biomechanical alignment, as well as the materials for fabrication. Communication with the orthotist,who will fabricate or fit the brace, is of utmost importance in order to obtain a good clinical result.

Psychology of Injury

Injury is more than physical; that is, the athlete must be psychologically ready for the demands of his or her sport. The most immediate emotional response at the point of injury is shock. It's degree may range from minor to significant, depending upon the severity of the injury. It is important to note that denial itself is an adaptive response that allows an individual to manage extreme emotional responses to situational stress. Many individuals assist athletes through the recovery process and can foster psychological readiness, but they can also identify those who are physically recovered but require more time or intervention to be fully prepared to return to competition. Thus, rehabilitation and recovery are not purely physical but also psychological.

Mental skills in sports are often viewed as part of an individual's personality and something that cannot be taught. Many physicians feel that injured athletes either have or do not have the mental toughness to progress through rehabilitation. Mental skills, however, can be learned. One example for this is to provide proper goal setting, which has very important role in sports rehabilitation, because they can enhance recovery from injury. Goal setting needs to be measurable and stated in behavioral terms. The research indicates that goals should be challenging and difficult, yet attainable. It is important for physicians to help them focus on short-term goals as a means to attain long-term goals. For example, to set daily and weekly goals in rehabilitation process which will end in long-term goal like returning to play after an injury. It is important for sports medicine physicians to assist patients in setting goals related to performance process rather than outcomes, such as returning to play.

Stages of Rehabilitation

Initial Stage of Rehabilitation

This phase lasts approximately 4-6 days. The body's first response to an injury is inflammation. It's main function is to defend the body against harmful substances, dispose of dead or dying tissue and to promote the renewal of normal tissue. The goals during the initial phase of the rehabilitation process include limitation of tissue damage, pain relief, control of the inflammatory response to injury, and protection of the affected anatomical area. The pathological events that take place immediately after the injury could lead to impairments such as muscle atrophy and weakness and limitation in the joint range of motion. These impairments result in functional losses, for example, inability to jump or lift an object. The extent of the functional loss may be influenced by the nature and timing of the therapeutic and rehabilitative intervention during the initial phase of the injury. If functional losses are severe or become permanent, the athlete now with a disability may be unable to participate in his/her sport.

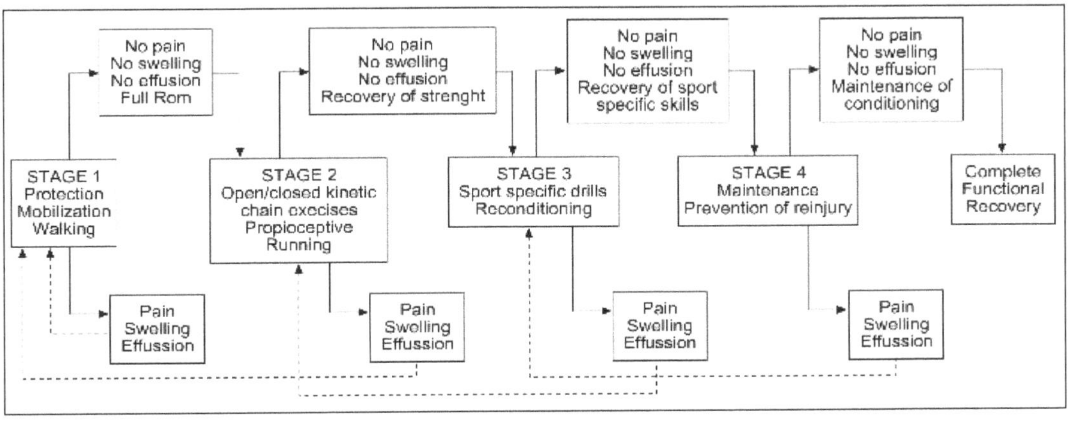

The physiotherapist is usually the professional in charge of this phase although the process may be started by a medical doctor.

Control Pain and Swelling

Primary treatment in initial phase of rehabilitation is RICE. It is the term that stands for Rest, Ice, Compression and Elevation. RICE can be used immediately and 24 to 48 hours after many muscle strains, ligament sprains, or other bruises and injuries.

Therapeutic modalities and medications are used to create an optimal environment for injury repair by limiting the inflammatory process and breaking the pain-spasm cycle. Use of any modality depends on the supervising physician's exercise prescription, as well as the injury site, and type and severity of injury. In some cases, a modality may be indicated and contraindicated for the same condition. For example, thermotherapy (heat therapy) may be contraindicated for tendinitis during the initial phase of the exercise program. However, once acute inflammation is controlled, heat therapy may be indicated. Frequent evaluation of the individual's progress is necessary to ensure that the appropriate modality is being used.

Despite the fact that rapid return to competition is crucial, rest is necessary to protect the damaged tissue from additional injury. Therefore, exercise involving the injured area is not recomended during this phase, although there are a few exceptions such as the tendinopathy protocols used to rehabilitate Achilles and patella tendon injuries.

However, it is important to realize that a quick return to function relies on the health of other body tissues.

The power, strength, and endurance of the musculoskeletal tissues and the function of the cardiorespiratory system must be maintained. Athlete needs to understands the reasons for following a particular treatment regime or exercise program, as well medical professional's advice should be sought before embarking on any regime as more harm can be done than good if carried out incorrectly.

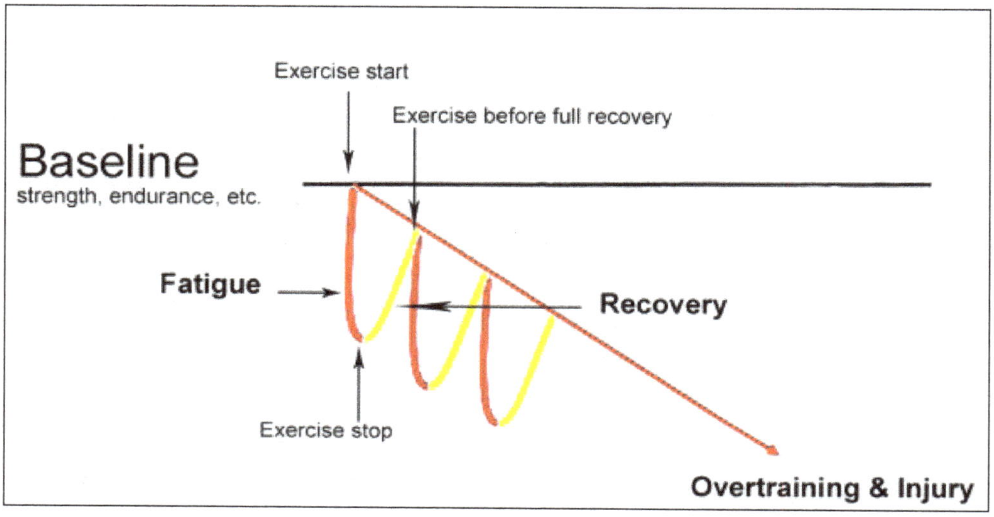

Active range of motion is performed under one's own control, while passive range of motion occurs when another person or device produces the movement. If movement of the injured limb is not contraindicated, isolated exercises that target areas proximal and distal to the injured area may be permissible provided that they do not stress the injured area. Examples include hip abduction and rotation exercises following knee injury or scapula stabilizing exercises following glenohumeral joint injury. Isometric exercises are used for strengthening when range of motion is restricted or needs to be avoided due to the fracture or acute inflammation of a joint. Otherwise, isotonic strengthening can begin within the painless arc of joint motion.

Intermediate Stage of Rehabilitation

This phase lasts from day 5 to 8-10 weeks. After the inflammatory phase, the body begins to repair the damaged tissue with similar tissue, but the resiliency of the new tissue is low. Repair of the weakened injury site can take up to eight weeks if the proper amount of restorative stress is applied, or longer if too much or too little stress is applied.

Joint ROM and Muscle Conditioning

The goals during the second phase of rehabilitation include the limitation of the impairment and the recovery from the functional losses. Early protected motion hastens the optimal alignment of collagen fibers and promotes improved tissue mobility. A number of physical modalities are used to enhance tissue healing. Exercise to regain flexibility, strength, endurance, balance, and coordination become the central component of the intervention. To the extent that these impairments and functional losses were minimized by early intervention, progress in this phase can be accelerated. Again, the maintenance of muscular and cardiorespiratory function remains essential for the uninjured areas of the body. The strength and conditioning professional has considerable expertise to offer the other members of the sports medicine team regarding selection of the appropriate activities.

Possible exercise forms during this phase include strengthening of the uninjured extremities and areas proximal and distal to the injury, aerobic and anaerobic exercise, and improving strength and neuromuscular control of the involved areas:

- Isometric exercise may be performed provided that it is pain free and otherwise indicated. Submaximal isometric exercise allows the athlete to maintain neuromuscular function and improve strength with movements performed at an intensity low enough that the newly formed collagen fibers are not disrupted.
- Isokinetic exercise can be an important aspect of strengthening following injury. This type of exercise uses equipment that provides resistance to movement at a given speed (e.g., 60°/s or 120°/s).
- Isotonic exercise involves movements with constant external resistance and the amount of force required to move the resistance varies, depending primarily on joint angle and the length of each agonist muscle. Isotonic exercise uses several different forms of resistance, including gravity (i.e., exercises performed without equipment, with gravitational effects as the only source of resistance), dumbbells, barbells, and weight-stack machines. The speed at which the movement occurs is controlled by the athlete; movement speed can be a program design variable, with more acute injuries calling for slower movement and the later phases of healing amenable to faster, more sport-specific movement.
- Specific types of exercises exist to improve neuromuscular control following injury and can be manipulated through alterations in surface stability, vision, and speed. Mini-trampolines, balance boards, and stability balls can be used to create unstable surfaces for upper and lower extremity training. Athletes can perform common activities such as squats and push-ups on uneven surfaces to improve neuromuscular control.
- Exercises may also be performed with eyes closed, thus removing visual input, to further challenge balance.

Finally, increasing the speed at which exercises are performed provides additional challenges to the system. Specifically controlling these variables within a controlled environment will allow the athlete to progress to more challenging exercises in the next stage of healing.

Advanced Stage of Rehabilitation

This phase begins at around 21 days and can continue for 6-12 months. The outcome of the previous phase is the replacement of damaged tissue with collagen fibers. After those fibers are laid down, the body can begin to remodel and strengthen the new tissue, allowing the athlete to gradually return to full activity. This phase of rehabilitation represents the start of the conditioning process needed to return to sports training and competition. Understanding the demands of the particular sport becomes essential as well as communication with the coach. This phase also represents an opportunity to identify and correct risk factors, thus reducing the possibility of re-injury.

Functional Training

The combination of clinic-based and sport-specific functional techniques will provide an individualized, sport-specific rehabilitation protocol for the athlete. Rehabilitation and reconditioning exercises must be functional to facilitate a return to competition. Examples of functional training include joint angle-specific strengthening, velocity-specific muscle activity, closed kinetic chain exercises, and exercises designed to further enhance neuromuscular control. Strengthening should transition from general exercises to sport-specific exercises designed to replicate movements common in given sports. Cross-training is encouraged, especially with activities that do not produce any symptoms from the injury.

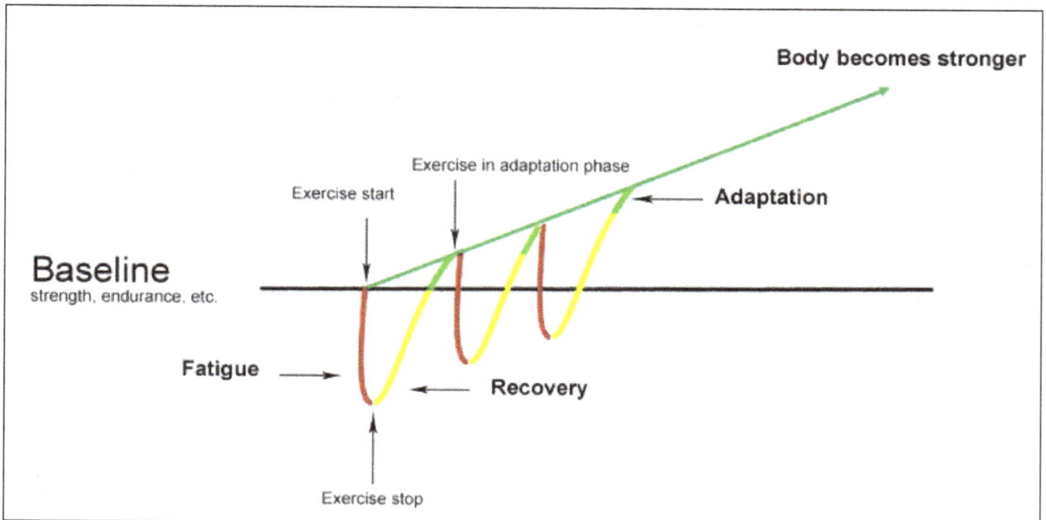

It is essential that the rehabilitation and training be sufficiently vigorous to prepare the injured tissue for the demands of the game. With each increase in activity, signs of recurring pain or weakness should trigger a slowdown or a reversal to a tolerable level of activity. The player will have returned to game during this phase and will have ceased physiotherapy or individual rehabilitation while this process is still continuing. Unrestricted sports activity is not allowed until all of these steps have been completed and full-effort sports-specific activity is tolerated without symptoms.

Return to Sport

At some point in the recovery process, athletes return to strength and conditioning programs and resume sport-specific activities in preparation for return to play. The transition is important for several reasons. First, although the athlete may have recovered in medical terms (ie, improvements in flexibility, range of motion, functional strength, pain, neuromuscular control, inflammation), preparation for competition requires the restoration of strength, power, speed, agility, and endurance at levels exhibited in sport.

Return to play is defined as the process of deciding when an injured or ill athlete may safely return to practice or competition. Early return to training and sport are considered sensible goals if the rate of return is based on the affected muscle, the severity of the injury and the position of the athlete.

Criteria for return to play must emphasize gradual return to sport-specific functional progressions. Sport-specific function occurs when the activations, motions and resultant forces are specific and efficient for the needs of that sport. Sport-specific functional rehabilitation should focus on restoration of the injured athlete's ability to have sport-specific physiology and biomechanics to interact optimally with the sport-specific demands. That means that they need to be replicated at the same speed, on the same surface and with the same level of fatigue to be truly effective.

Once a athlete has been medically cleared to return-to-play there are some fundamental steps that need to be followed:

- The athlete has to fulfill the fitness standards of the team he is returning to.
- The athlete needs to pass some skill specific tests applicable to his playing position.
- The player may then begin practicing with the team.
- Exposure to the match situation should be gradual, with the match time gradually increasing.

There are simple guidelines which need to be developed by each team with contributions and support from each member of the medical team.

Monitoring

Regarding these aspects from the text above, there are several problems: are all the mechanic parameters of the performance (force, velocity, power) regained at that time?

Are there any ways to conduct the rehabilitation program in order to obtain better parameters and so the return to the sports activity to be safely done? Which could be the most suitable evaluation methods in order to be sure about the athletes well-training?

Monitoring athlete well-being is essential to guide training and to detect any progression towards negative health outcomes and associated poor performance. Objective (performance, physiological, biochemical) and subjective measures (mood disturbance, perceived stress and recovery and symptoms of stress) are all options for athlete monitoring. Appropriate load monitoring can aid in determining whether an athlete is adapting to a training program and in minimizing the risk of developing non-functional overreaching, illness, and/or injury.

In order to gain an understanding of the training load and its effect on the athlete, a number of potential markers are available for use. There are a number of external load quantifying and monitoring tools, such as power output measuring devices, time-motion analysis, as well as internal load unit measures, including perception of effort, heart rate, blood lactate, and training impulse. Other monitoring tools used by high-performance programs include heart rate recovery, neuromuscular function, biochemical/hormonal/immunological assessments, questionnaires and diaries, psychomotor speed, and sleep quality and quantity. Coaching staffs and administrative personnel must work to ensure that care can be provided at all points of the rehabilitation process, especially when funding dictates the need to hire personnel capable of addressing injuries at multiple levels. A clear understanding of the injury and of the interventions from each provider is vital to an efficient and successful return to play.

Appropriate monitoring of training load can provide important information to athletes and coaches; however, monitoring systems should be intuitive, provide efficient data analysis and interpretation, and enable efficient reporting of simple, yet scientifically valid, feedback. If accurate and easy-to-interpret feedback is provided to the athlete and coach, load monitoring can result in enhanced knowledge of training responses, aid in the design of training programs, provide a further avenue for communication between support staff and athletes and coaches and ultimately enhance an athlete's performance.

References

- Physical-medicine-and-rehabilitation, science: britannica.com, Retrieved 17 February , 2020
- 8-types-of-physical-medicine-and-rehabilitation: guidedoc.com, Retrieved 13 July, 2020
- Rehabilitation: medlineplus.gov, Retrieved 28 April, 2020
- Rehabilitation-in-Sport: physio-pedia.com, Retrieved 19 May, 2020

Specializations in Physical Medicine 2

- Sports Medicine
- Pain Management
- Neuromuscular Medicine
- Hospice and Palliative Medicine
- Postural Restoration

There are various sub-specializations that fall under the domain of physical medicine such as sports medicine, neuromuscular medicine, hospice and palliative medicine, etc. This chapter closely examines these sub-specializations of physical medicine to provide an extensive understanding of the subject.

Sports Medicine

Sports medicine, also known as sports and exercise medicine (SEM), is a branch of medicine that deals with physical fitness and the treatment and prevention of injuries related to sports and exercise The goal of a sports medicine is to help people engage in exercise safely and effectively in order to achieve their training goals.

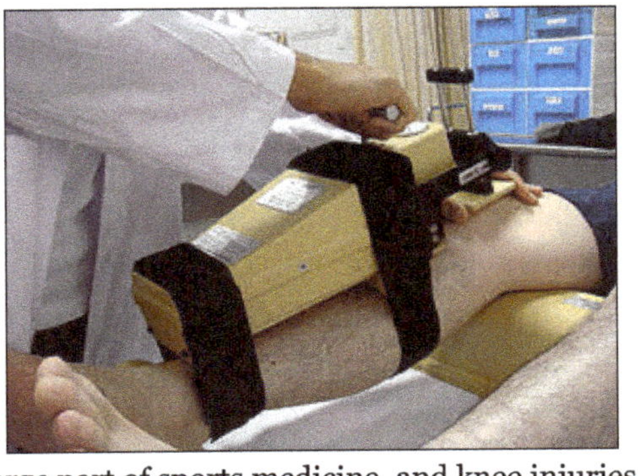

Orthopaedics is a large part of sports medicine, and knee injuries a common theme.
Here a subject is having the anterior-posterior laxity of his knee tested.

Sports medicine specialists treat a wide range of physical conditions, including acute traumas such as fractures, sprains, strains, and dislocations. They also treat chronic overuse injuries, including tendonitis, degenerative diseases, and overtraining syndrome.

Sports medicine combines general medical education with the specific principles of sports science, exercise physiology, orthopedics, biomechanics, sports nutrition, and even sports psychology.

A sports medicine team may involve medical and non-medical specialists, including physicians, surgeons, athletic trainers, sports psychologists, physical therapists, nutritionists, coaches, and personal trainers.

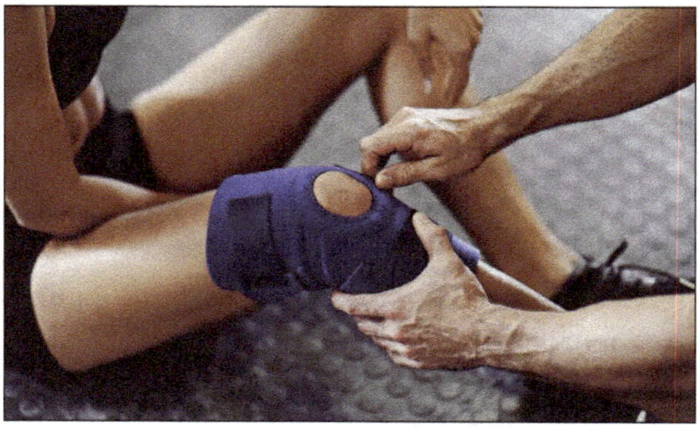

Sports Medicine Specialists

A sports medicine specialist focuses on the medical, therapeutic, and functional aspects of exercise and works directly with athletes to improve their overall sports performance.

The title of "sports medicine specialist" does not necessarily mean the specialist is a physician. It can be applied to any number of disciplines for which sports medical practices are used.

Sports medicine is not a medical specialty in and of itself. Rather, it implies additional training focused on the medical aspects of sports and exercise after foundational certification has first been achieved. Non-medical professionals involved in sports medicine include:

- Physical therapists who help people recover from injuries.
- Certified athletic trainers who provide rehabilitative programs to help athletes regain strength and prevent future injury.
- Nutritionists who assist with weight management and nutrition in conjunction with physical training or recovery.

Sports Medicine Physicians

Sports medicine physicians are medical doctors who specialized in the diagnosis and treatment of sports- or exercise-related injuries and illness. While many sports medicine physicians work exclusively with athletes, the majority will treat anyone who needs treatment after a sports injury.

Most sports medicine physicians are first certified in family practice, emergency medicine, pediatrics, internal medicine, or orthopedics before embarking on a two-year fellowship in sports medicine. Upon completion, many will earn a Certificate of Added Qualifications (CAQ) in Sports Medicine from the American Board of Family Medicine.

Most sports medicine physicians deal with non-operative musculoskeletal conditions. Others are orthopedic surgeons who have decided to focus their practice on the surgical treatment of sports injuries.

Beyond muscle, bones, and joint injuries, a sports medicine physician will be qualified to treat any number of other associated conditions, including:

- Concussion and other head injuries.
- Chronic or acute illnesses (such as asthma, diabetes, or hypertension).
- Nutrition, supplements, ergogenic aids, and performance issues.
- Injury prevention.
- "Return to play" decisions in sick or injured athletes.

Generally speaking, sports medicine physicians will tend to earn higher incomes than their non-specialist counterparts.

Sports Psychologists

Sports psychology is a specific branch of psychology that focuses on the mental and emotional needs of athletes and sports enthusiasts. The field of sports psychology is becoming more prominent and accepted among athletes. It is not uncommon for professional sports teams to employ a full-time psychologist to help prepare the team for competition or to overcome emotional challenges that can impede performance.

Because athletes face unique stresses, a sports psychologist can help regulate anxiety and improve focus in a way that is specific to their sport. They will use a variety of psychology tools and skills (including psychotherapy, stress management, and goal-setting) to help the athlete maintain a strong emotional balance during competition or the recovery from a severe sports injury.

Sports Science Specialists

Sports science, also referred to as exercise science, is the focused study of the principals of physiology, anatomy, and psychology as they relate to human movement and physical activity. As a discipline, exercise science is still in its infancy and primarily focused on clinical research (including physiological responses to exercise, comparative effectiveness of exercise techniques, and the impact of performance-enhancing drugs and supplements).

Pain Management

Pain management, pain medicine, pain control or algiatry, is a branch of medicine employing an interdisciplinary approach for easing the suffering and improving the quality of life of those living with chronic pain. The typical pain management team includes medical practitioners, pharmacists, clinical psychologists, physiotherapists, occupational therapists, physician assistants, nurses. The team may also include other mental health specialists and massage therapists. Pain sometimes resolves promptly once the underlying trauma or pathology has healed, and is treated by one practitioner, with drugs such as analgesics and (occasionally) anxiolytics. Effective management of chronic (long-term) pain, however, frequently requires the coordinated efforts of the pain management team. Effective pain management does not mean total eradication of all pain.

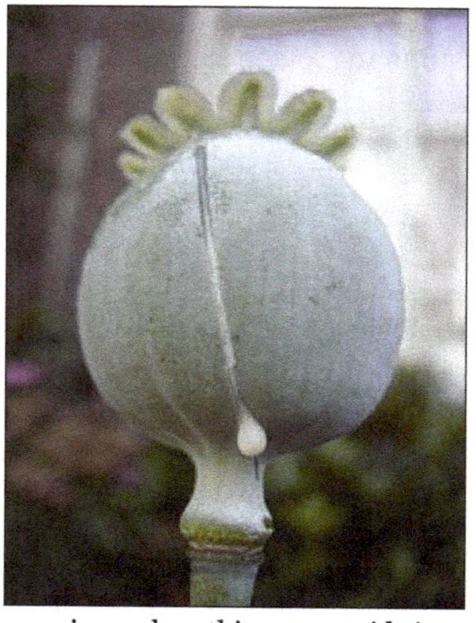

Opium poppies such as this one provide ingredients for the class of analgesics called opiates.

Medicine treats injuries and diseases to support and speed healing, and it treats distressing symptoms such as pain to relieve suffering during treatment, healing, and dying. When a painful injury or pathology is resistant to treatment and persists, when pain persists after the injury or pathology has healed, and when medical science cannot identify the cause of pain, the task of medicine is to relieve suffering. Treatment approaches to chronic pain include pharmacological measures, such as analgesics, antidepressants and anticonvulsants, interventional procedures, physical therapy, physical exercise, application of ice and heat, and psychological measures, such as biofeedback and cognitive behavioral therapy.

Uses

Pain can have many causes and there are many possible treatments for it. In the nursing profession, one common definition of pain is any problem that is "whatever the experiencing person says it is, existing whenever the experiencing person says it does". Different sorts of pain management address different sorts of pain.

Pain management includes patient communication about the pain problem. To define the pain problem, a health care provider will likely ask questions such as these:

- How intense is the pain?
- How does the pain feel?
- Where is the pain?
- What, if anything, makes the pain lessen?
- What, if anything, makes the pain increase?
- When did the pain start?

After asking questions such as these, the health care provider will have a description of the pain. Pain management will then be used to address that pain.

Adverse Effects

There are many types of pain management, and each of them have their own benefits, drawbacks, and limits.

A common difficulty in pain management is communication. People experiencing pain may have difficulty recognizing or describing what they feel and how intense it is. Health care providers and patients may have difficulty communicating with each other about how pain responds to treatments. There is a continuing risk in many types of pain management for the patient to take treatment which is less effective than needed or which causes other difficulty and side effects. Some treatments for pain can be harmful if overused. A goal of pain management for the patient and their health care provider to identify the amount of treatment which addresses the pain but which is not too much treatment.

Another problem with pain management is that pain is the body's natural way of communicating a problem. Pain is supposed to resolve as the body heals itself with time and pain management. Sometimes pain management covers a problem, and the patient might be less aware that they need treatment for a deeper problem.

Physical Approach

Physical Medicine and Rehabilitation

Physical medicine and rehabilitation employs diverse physical techniques such as thermal agents and electrotherapy, as well as therapeutic exercise and behavioral therapy, alone or in tandem with interventional techniques and conventional pharmacotherapy to treat pain, usually as part of an interdisciplinary or multidisciplinary program. The Center for Disease Control recommends that physical therapy and exercise can be prescribed as a positive alternative to opioids for decreasing one's pain in multiple injuries, illnesses, or diseases. This can include chronic low back pain, osteoarthritis of the hip and knee, or fibromyalgia. Exercise alone or with other rehabilitation disciplines (such as psychologically based approaches) can have a positive effect on reducing pain. In addition to improving pain, exercise also can improve one's well-being and general health.

Exercise Interventions

Physical activity interventions, such as tai chi, yoga and Pilates, promote harmony of the mind and body through total body awareness. These ancient practices incorporate breathing techniques, meditation and a wide variety of movements, while training the body to perform functionally by increasing strength, flexibility, and range of motion. Physical activity and exercise may improve chronic pain (pain lasting more than 12 weeks), and overall quality of life, while minimizing the need for pain medications.

TENS

Transcutaneous electrical nerve stimulation has been found to be ineffective for lower back pain, however, it might help with diabetic neuropathy.

Acupuncture

Acupuncture involves the insertion and manipulation of needles into specific points on the body to relieve pain or for therapeutic purposes. An analysis of the 13 highest quality studies of pain treatment with acupuncture, published in January 2009 in the *British Medical Journal,* was unable to quantify the difference in the effect on pain of real, sham and no acupuncture.

Light Therapy

Research has not found evidence that light therapy such as low level laser therapy is an effective therapy for relieving low back pain.

Interventional Procedures

Interventional procedures - typically used for chronic back pain - include epidural steroid injections, facet joint injections, neurolytic blocks, spinal cord stimulators and intrathecal drug delivery system implants.

Pulsed radiofrequency, neuromodulation, direct introduction of medication and nerve ablation may be used to target either the tissue structures and organ/systems responsible for persistent nociception or the nociceptors from the structures implicated as the source of chronic pain.

An intrathecal pump used to deliver very small quantities of medications directly to the spinal fluid. This is similar to epidural infusions used in labour and postoperatively. The major differences are that it is much more common for the drug to be delivered into the spinal fluid (intrathecal) rather than epidurally, and the pump can be fully implanted under the skin.

A spinal cord stimulator is an implantable medical device that creates electric impulses and applies them near the dorsal surface of the spinal cord provides a paresthesia ("tingling") sensation that alters the perception of pain by the patient.

Psychological Approach

Cognitive Behavioral Therapy

Cognitive behavioral therapy (CBT) for pain helps patients with pain to understand the relationship between one's physiology (e.g., pain and muscle tension), thoughts, emotions, and behaviors. A main goal in treatment is cognitive restructuring to encourage helpful thought patterns, targeting a behavioral activation of healthy activities such as regular exercise and pacing. Lifestyle changes are also trained to improve sleep patterns and to develop better coping skills for pain and other stressors using various techniques (e.g., relaxation, diaphragmatic breathing, and even biofeedback).

Studies have demonstrated the usefulness of cognitive behavioral therapy in the management of chronic low back pain, producing significant decreases in physical and psychosocial disability. CBT is significantly more effective than standard care in treatment of people with body-wide pain, like fibromyalgia. Evidence for the usefulness of CBT in the management of adult chronic pain is generally poorly understood, due partly to the proliferation of techniques of doubtful quality, and the poor quality of reporting in clinical trials. The crucial content of individual interventions has not been isolated and the important contextual elements, such as therapist training and development of treatment manuals, have not been determined. The widely varying nature of the resulting data makes useful systematic review and meta-analysis within the field very difficult.

In 2012, a systematic review of randomized controlled trials (RCTs) evaluated the clinical effectiveness of psychological therapies for the management of adult chronic pain (excluding headaches). There is no evidence that behaviour therapy (BT) is effective for reducing this type of pain, however BT may be useful for improving a persons mood immediately after treatment. This improvement appears to be small, and is short term in duration. CBT may have a small positive short-term effect on pain immediately following treatment. CBT may also have a small effect on reducing disability and potential catastrophizing that may be associated with adult chronic pain. These benefits do not appear to last very long following the therapy. CBT may contribute towards improving the mood of an adult who experiences chronic pain, and there is a possibility that this benefit may be maintained for longer periods of time.

For children and adolescents, a review of RCTs evaluating the effectiveness of psychological therapy for the management of chronic and recurrent pain found that psychological treatments are effective in reducing pain when people under 18 years old have headaches. This beneficial effect may be maintained for at least three months following the therapy. Psychological treatments may also improve pain control for children or adolescents who experience pain not related to headaches. It is not known if psychological therapy improves a child or adolescents mood and the potential for disability related to their chronic pain.

Hypnosis

A 2007 review of 13 studies found evidence for the efficacy of hypnosis in the reduction of pain in some conditions, though the number of patients enrolled in the studies was small, bringing up issues of power to detect group differences, and most lacked credible controls for placebo and expectation. The authors concluded that "although the findings provide support for the general applicability of hypnosis in the treatment of chronic pain, considerably more research will be needed to fully determine the effects of hypnosis for different chronic-pain conditions."

Hypnosis has reduced the pain of some noxious medical procedures in children and adolescents, and in clinical trials addressing other patient groups it has significantly reduced pain compared to no treatment or some other non-hypnotic interventions. However, no studies have compared hypnosis to a convincing placebo, so the pain reduction may be due to patient expectation (the "placebo effect"). The effects of self hypnosis on chronic pain are roughly comparable to those of progressive muscle relaxation.

Mindfulness Meditation

A meta-analysis of studies that used techniques centered around the concept of mindfulness, concluded, "Findings suggest that MBIs decrease the intensity of pain for chronic pain patients."

Medications

The World Health Organization (WHO) recommends a *pain ladder* for managing analgesia. It was first described for use in cancer pain, but it can be used by medical professionals as a general principle when dealing with analgesia for any type of pain. In the treatment of chronic pain, whether due to malignant or benign processes, the three-step WHO Analgesic Ladder provides guidelines for selecting the kind and stepping up the amount of analgesia. The exact medications recommended will vary with the country and the individual treatment center, but the following gives an example of the WHO approach to treating chronic pain with medications. If, at any point, treatment fails to provide adequate pain relief, then the doctor and patient move onto the next step.

Table: Common types of pain and typical drug management.

Pain type	Typical initial drug treatment	Comments
Headache	Paracetamol/acetaminophen, NSAIDs	Doctor consultation is appropriate if headaches are severe, persistent, accompanied by fever, vomiting, or speech or balance problems; self-medication should be limited to two weeks.
Migraine	Paracetamol, NSAIDs	Triptans are used when the others do not work, or when migraines are frequent or severe.
Menstrual cramps	NSAIDs	Some NSAIDs are marketed for cramps, but any NSAID would work.
Minor trauma, such as a bruise, abrasions, sprain	Paracetamol, NSAIDs	Opioids not recommended.
Severe trauma, such as a wound, burn, bone fracture, or severe sprain	Opioids	More than two weeks of pain requiring opioid treatment is unusual.
Strain or pulled muscle	NSAIDs, muscle relaxants	If inflammation is involved, NSAIDs may work better; short-term use only.
Minor pain after surgery	Paracetamol, NSAIDs	Opioids rarely needed.
Severe pain after surgery	Opioids	Combinations of opioids may be prescribed if pain is severe.
Muscle ache	Paracetamol, NSAIDs	If inflammation involved, NSAIDs may work better.
Toothache or pain from dental procedures	Paracetamol, NSAIDs	This should be short term use; opioids may be necessary for severe pain.
Kidney stone pain	Paracetamol, NSAIDs, opioids	Opioids usually needed if pain is severe.
Pain due to heartburn or gastroesophageal reflux disease	Antacid, H2 antagonist, proton-pump inhibitor	Heartburn lasting more than a week requires medical attention; aspirin and NSAIDs should be avoided.

Chronic back pain	Paracetamol, NSAIDs	Opioids may be necessary if other drugs do not control pain and pain is persistent.
Osteoarthritis pain	Paracetamol, NSAIDs	Medical attention is recommended if pain persists.
Fibromyalgia	Antidepressant, anticonvulsant	Evidence suggests that opioids are not effective in treating fibromyalgia.

Mild Pain

Paracetamol (acetaminophen), or a nonsteroidal anti-inflammatory drug (NSAID) such as ibuprofen.

Mild to Moderate Pain

Paracetamol, an NSAID and/or paracetamol in a combination product with a weak opioid such as tramadol, may provide greater relief than their separate use. Also a combination of opioid with acetaminophen can be frequently used such as Percocet, Vicodin, or Norco.

Moderate to Severe Pain

When treating moderate to severe pain, the type of the pain, acute or chronic, needs to be considered. The type of pain can result in different medications being prescribed. Certain medications may work better for acute pain, others for chronic pain, and some may work equally well on both. Acute pain medication is for rapid onset of pain such as from an inflicted trauma or to treat post-operative pain. Chronic pain medication is for alleviating long-lasting, ongoing pain.

Morphine is the gold standard to which all narcotics are compared. Semi-synthetic derivatives of morphine such as hydromorphone (Dilaudid), oxymorphone (Numorphan, Opana), nicomorphine (Vilan), hydromorphinol and others vary in such ways as duration of action, side effect profile and milligramme potency. Fentanyl has the benefit of less histamine release and thus fewer side effects. It can also be administered via transdermal patch which is convenient for chronic pain management. In addition to the intrathecal patch and injectable Sublimaze, the FDA has approved various immediate release fentanyl products for breakthrough cancer pain (Actiq/OTFC/Fentora/Onsolis/Subsys/Lazanda/Abstral). Oxycodone is used across the Americas and Europe for relief of serious chronic pain; its main slow-release formula is known as OxyContin, and short-acting tablets, capsules, syrups and ampules are available making it suitable for acute intractable pain or breakthrough pain. Diamorphine, methadone and buprenorphine are used less frequently. Pethidine, known in North America as meperidine, is not recommended for pain management due to its low potency, short duration of action, and toxicity associated with repeated use. Pentazocine, dextromoramide and dipipanone are also not recommended in new patients except for acute pain where other analgesics are not tolerated or are inappropriate, for pharmacological and misuse-related reasons. In some countries potent synthetics such as piritramide and ketobemidone are used for severe pain, and tapentadol is a newer agent introduced in the last decade.

For moderate pain, tramadol, codeine, dihydrocodeine, and hydrocodone are used, with nicocodeine, ethylmorphine and propoxyphene and dextropropoxyphene less commonly.

Drugs of other types can be used to help opioids combat certain types of pain, for example, amitriptyline is prescribed for chronic muscular pain in the arms, legs, neck and lower back with an opiate, or sometimes without it and with an NSAID. While opiates are often used in the management of chronic pain, high doses are associated with an increased risk of opioid overdose.

Opioids

According to the National Institutes of Health, studies have shown that properly managed medical use of opioid analgesic compounds (taken exactly as prescribed) is safe, can manage pain effectively, and rarely causes addiction.

Opioid medications can provide short, intermediate or long acting analgesia depending upon the specific properties of the medication and whether it is formulated as an extended release drug. Opioid medications may be administered orally, by injection, via nasal mucosa or oral mucosa, rectally, transdermally, intravenously, epidurally and intrathecally. In chronic pain conditions that are opioid responsive a combination of a long-acting (OxyContin, MS Contin, Opana ER, Exalgo and Methadone) or extended release medication is often prescribed in conjunction with a shorter-acting medication (oxycodone, morphine or hydromorphone) for breakthrough pain, or exacerbations.

Most opioid treatment used by patients outside of healthcare settings is oral (tablet, capsule or liquid), but suppositories and skin patches can be prescribed. An opioid injection is rarely needed for patients with chronic pain.

Although opioids are strong analgesics, they do not provide complete analgesia regardless of whether the pain is acute or chronic in origin. Opioids are efficacious analgesics in chronic malignant pain and modestly effective in nonmalignant pain management. However, there are associated adverse effects, especially during the commencement or change in dose. When opioids are used for prolonged periods drug tolerance, chemical dependency, diversion and addiction may occur.

Clinical guidelines for prescribing opioids for chronic pain have been issued by the American Pain Society and the American Academy of Pain Medicine. Included in these guidelines is the importance of assessing the patient for the risk of substance abuse, misuse, or addiction; a personal or family history of substance abuse is the strongest predictor of aberrant drug-taking behavior. Physicians who prescribe opioids should integrate this treatment with any psychotherapeutic intervention the patient may be receiving. The guidelines also recommend monitoring not only the pain but also the level of functioning and the achievement of therapeutic goals. The prescribing physician should be suspicious of abuse when a patient reports a reduction in pain but has no accompanying improvement in function or progress in achieving identified goals.

Commonly-used long-acting opioids and their parent compound:

- OxyContin (oxycodone).
- Hydromorph Contin (hydromorphone).
- MS Contin (morphine).
- M-Eslon (morphine).
- Exalgo (hydromorphone).
- Opana ER (oxymorphone).
- Duragesic (fentanyl).
- Nucynta ER (tapentadol).
- Metadol/Methadose (methadone)*.
- Hysingla ER (hydrocodone bitartrate).
- Zohydro ER (hydrocodone bicarbonate).

*Methadone can be used for either treatment of opioid addiction/detoxification when taken once daily or as a pain medication usually administered on an every 12-hour or 8-hour dosing interval.

*The long-lasting version of OxyContin was a major contributor of the opioid epidemic.

Nonsteroidal Anti-inflammatory Drugs

The other major group of analgesics are nonsteroidal anti-inflammatory drugs (NSAID). They work by inhibiting the release of prostaglandins, which cause inflammatory pain. Acetaminophen/paracetamol is not always included in this class of medications. However, acetaminophen may be administered as a single medication or in combination with other analgesics (both NSAIDs and opioids). The alternatively prescribed NSAIDs such as ketoprofen and piroxicam have limited benefit in chronic pain disorders and with long-term use are associated with significant adverse effects. The use of selective NSAIDs designated as selective COX-2 inhibitors have significant cardiovascular and cerebrovascular risks which have limited their utilization. Common NSAIDs include aspirin, ibuprofen, and naproxen.

Antidepressants and Antiepileptic Drugs

Some antidepressant and antiepileptic drugs are used in chronic pain management and act primarily within the pain pathways of the central nervous system, though peripheral mechanisms have been attributed as well. They are generally used to treat nerve brain that results from injury to the nervous system. Neuropathy can be due to chronic high blood sugar levels (diabetic neuropathy); and viruses, such as shingles; phantom limb pain; or post-stroke pain. These mechanisms vary and in general are more effective in neuropathic pain disorders as well as complex regional pain syndrome. A common anti-epileptic drug is gabapentin, and an example of an antidepressant would be amitriptyline.

Cannabinoids

Chronic pain is one of the most commonly cited reasons for the use of medical marijuana. A 2012 Canadian survey of participants in their medical marijuana program found that 84% of respondents reported using medical marijuana for the management of pain.

Evidence of medical marijuana's pain mitigating effects is generally conclusive. Detailed in a 1999 report by the Institute of Medicine, "the available evidence from animal and human studies indicates that cannabinoids can have a substantial analgesic effect". In a 2013 review study published in *Fundamental & Clinical Pharmacology*, various studies were cited in demonstrating that cannabinoids exhibit comparable effectiveness to opioids in models of acute pain and even greater effectiveness in models of chronic pain.

Other Analgesics

Other drugs are often used to help analgesics combat various types of pain, and parts of the overall pain experience, and are hence called analgesic adjuvant medications. Gabapentin—an anti-epileptic—not only exerts effects alone on neuropathic pain, but can potentiate opiates. While perhaps not prescribed as such, other drugs such as Tagamet (cimetidine) and even simple grapefruit juice may also potentiate opiates, by inhibiting CYP450 enzymes in the liver, thereby slowing metabolism of the drug. In addition, orphenadrine, cyclobenzaprine, trazodone and other drugs with anticholinergic properties are useful in conjunction with opioids for neuropathic pain. Orphenadrine and cyclobenzaprine are also muscle relaxants, and therefore particularly useful in painful musculoskeletal conditions.

Neuromuscular Medicine

Neuromuscular medicine is subspecialty of neurology and physiatry that focuses the diagnosis and treatment of neuromuscular diseases. The field encompasses issues related to both diagnosis and medical treatment of these conditions, as well as relevant rehabilitation interventions to optimize the quality of life of individuals with these conditions. This field encompasses disorders that impact both adults and children. Neuromuscular disease can be caused by autoimmune disorders, genetic/hereditary disorders such as channelopathies, or neurodegenerative diseases. Because they frequently have no cure, the focus is managing the condition to provide improvements in the patients quality. Rehabilitation robotics is a new frontier for neurological rehabilitation treatments.

Diagnostic Tools

The tools used to diagnose neuromuscular disorders include nerve and muscle biopsies, electromyography, nerve conduction studies, and molecular and genetic tests.

Hospice and Palliative Medicine

Hospice and palliative medicine is a formal subspecialty of medicine in the United States that focuses on symptom management, relief of suffering and end-of-life care.

In 2006, hospice and palliative medicine was officially recognized by the American Board of Medical Specialties, and is *co-sponsored* by:

- The American Boards of Internal Medicine.
- Anesthesiology.
- Family Medicine.
- Physical Medicine and Rehabilitation.
- Psychiatry and Neurology.
- Surgery.
- Pediatrics.
- Emergency Medicine.
- Radiology.
- Obstetrics and Gynecology.

Physicians who complete a residency in one of the *co-sponsoring* specialties are then eligible for further training in an ACGME-approved Hospice and Palliative Medicine fellowship program, after which they must pass the official examination to be board-certified in the subspecialty.

In 2007, the American Osteopathic Association Bureau of Osteopathic Specialists approved a Certificate of Added Qualifications (CAQ) in *hospice and palliative medicine.* By 2012 participants are the American Osteopathic Boards of:

- Internal Medicine.
- Family Medicine.
- Neurology and Psychiatry.
- Physical Medicine and Rehabilitation.

Candidates are eligible for CAQ certification after achieving board-certification following an American Osteopathic Association-approved residency.

Physicians in this subspecialty have advanced knowledge and skills to prevent and relieve the suffering experienced by patients with life-limiting, life-threatening and terminal illnesses. This specialist has expertise in the assessment of patients with advanced disease and catastrophic injury, the relief of distressing symptoms, the coordination of interdisciplinary patient and family-centered care in diverse settings, the use of specialized care systems including hospice, the management of the imminently dying patient; and legal and ethical decision making in end-of-life care. They work with an interdisciplinary hospice or palliative care team to maximize quality of life while addressing physical, psychological, social and spiritual needs of both patients and family members throughout the course of the disease, including through the dying process and subsequent bereavement. This care can occur within or outside of a formal hospice or palliative care team.

The American Academy of Hospice and Palliative Medicine (AAHPM) is the leading professional organization for physicians subspecializing in hospice and palliative medicine in North America. The International Association for Hospice and Palliative Care is the major professional organization devoted to the global spread of hospice and palliative medicine.

Postural Restoration

Postural Restoration (PRI) is a form of physical therapy treatment that encompasses the entire body. The main focus of the treatment is identifying and correcting common postural patterns found in the human body. A Postural Restoration Physical Therapist is trained to recognize, assess and treat biomechanical asymmetries that develop due to restricted motion in the body. Postural Restoration is an effective treatment approach for most musculoskeletal problems typically seen in physical therapy.

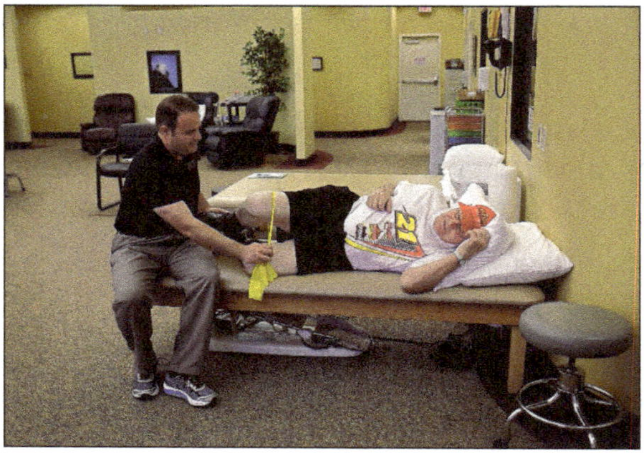

Postural Restoration Treatment Programs

Treatment programs are designed to address these specific asymmetries and restore more symmetrical, efficient motion. Central to treatment is breathing education. Patients will often breathe shallow or more into one lung. Poor breathing not only greatly affects body system function from a medical standpoint, but it limits proper rib cage and spine movement.

Each patient will be given an individualized treatment program allowing the patient to practice and learn techniques in the home. This allows ribs to move without restriction thus allowing the spine to rotate and joints move with less restriction.

As patients improve with these techniques, they will often experience greater freedom of movement, improved performance, and decreased pain.

Benefits

- Chronic Pain.
- Balance Disturbance/Falls.
- Difficulties with Walking or Running.
- Dizziness/Vertigo.
- Back, Hip or Sciatica Pain.
- SI Joint Sprains/Strains.
- Bursitis.
- Knee Pain.
- Foot Pain.

- Headaches/Neck Pain.
- Fibromyalgia/Pain Management.
- Difficulties with Breathing.
- Athletic Performance Issues.
- Scoliosis.
- Incontinence.
- Osteoporosis.
- Arthritis.
- Visual Deficits.
- Traumatic Brain Injury.
- Spinal Cord Injuries.
- Stroke/CVA.

References

- Sports-medicine-4014645: verywellfit.com, Retrieved 18 April, 2020
- Main CJ, Spanswick CC (2000). Pain management: an interdisciplinary approach. Churchill Livingstone. ISBN 978-0-443-05683-3
- Kraker, Jessica; a. Zivkovic, Sasa (2011). "Autoimmune Neuromuscular Disorders". Current Neuropharmacology. 9 (3): 400–8. doi:10.2174/157015911796558000. PMC 3151594. PMID 22379454
- Postural-restoration: balancemobilitytherapy.com, Retrieved 28 February, 2020

Sports Injuries and their Treatment

3

- Shin Splints
- Tennis Elbow
- Achilles Tendon Rupture
- Patellar Tendinitis
- Patellar Dislocation
- Climbing Injuries
- Rehabilitation in Spinal Cord Injury
- Exertional Rhabdomyolysis
- Rotator Cuff Tendinitis
- Lumbar Spine Pain
- Sports Concussion
- Ankle Sprains
- Hamstring Strain
- Plantar Fasciitis
- Meniscus Tear
- Calf Strain
- Rehabilitation of Ankle and Foot Injuries in Athletes

Sports injuries can occur due to overtraining, lack of conditioning, improper form and technique, etc. Some common injuries are shin splints, tennis elbow, Achilles tendon rupture, rotator cuff tendinitis, lumbar spine pain, etc. The topics elaborated in this chapter will help in gaining a better perspective of the sports injuries and treatment.

Shin Splints

The term "shin splints" describes pain felt along the front of your lower leg, at the shin bone. This pain concentrates in the lower leg between the knee and ankle. Shin splints frequently affect people who engage in moderate to heavy physical activity. You may be more likely to develop shin splints if you participate in strenuous physical activities or stop-start sports such as tennis, racquetball, soccer, or basketball.

Sometimes the pain of shin splints can be so intense that you must stop the activity. Shin splints is a cumulative stress disorder. Repeated pounding and stress on the bones, muscles, and joints of the lower legs prevents your body from being able to naturally repair and restore itself.

Causes of Shin Splints

The pain associated with shin splints results from excessive amounts of force on the shin bone and the tissues attaching the shin bone to the muscles surrounding it. The excessive force causes the muscles to swell and increases the pressure against the bone, leading to pain and inflammation.

Shin splints can also result from stress reactions to bone fractures. The constant pounding can cause minute cracks in the bones of the leg. The body can repair the cracks if given time to rest. However, if the body doesn't get time to rest, the tiny cracks can result in a complete fracture or a stress fracture.

People on Risk for Shin Splints

Various activities and physical attributes can put you at risk of getting shin splints. Risk factors include:

- An anatomical abnormality (such as flat foot syndrome).
- Muscle weakness in the thighs or buttocks.
- Lack of flexibility.
- Improper training techniques.
- Running downhill.
- Running on a slanted surface or uneven terrain.
- Running on hard surfaces like concrete.
- Using inappropriate or worn-out shoes for running or working out.
- Participating in sports that have fast stops and starts (like soccer or downhill skiing).

Shin splints are also more likely to occur when your leg muscles and tendons are tired. Women, people with flat feet or rigid arches, athletes, military recruits, and dancers all have an increased likelihood of developing shin splints.

Symptoms of Shin Splints

People with shin splints will experience some of the following symptoms:

- A dull ache in the front part of the lower leg.
- Pain that develops during exercise.
- Pain on either side of the shin bone.
- Muscle pain.
- Pain along the inner part of the lower leg.
- Tenderness or soreness along the inner part of the lower leg.
- Swelling in the lower leg (usually mild, if present).
- Numbness and weakness in the feet.

Tennis Elbow

Tennis elbow, also known as lateral epicondylitis, is a condition in which the outer part of the elbow becomes painful and tender. The pain may also extend into the back of the forearm and grip strength may be weak. Onset of symptoms is generally gradual. Golfer's elbow is a similar condition that affects the inside of the elbow.

It is due to excessive use of the muscles of the back of the forearm. Typically this occurs as a result of work or sports, classically racquet sports. The diagnosis is typically based on the symptoms with medical imaging used to rule out other potential causes. It is more likely if pain increases when a subject tries to bend back the wrist when the wrist is held in a neutral position. It is classified as a chronic tendinosis, not a tendinitis.

Treatment involves decreasing activities that bring on the symptoms together with physical therapy. Pain medications such as NSAIDS or acetaminophen may be used. A brace over the upper forearm may also be helpful. If the condition does not improve corticosteroid injections or surgery may be recommended. Many people get better within one month to two years.

About 2% of people are affected. Those 30 to 50 years old are most commonly affected. The condition was initially described in 1873. The name "lawn tennis elbow" first came into use for the condition in 1882.

Signs and Symptoms

- Pain on the outer part of the elbow (lateral epicondyle).

- Point tenderness over the lateral epicondyle—a prominent part of the bone on the outside of the elbow.
- Pain from gripping and movements of the wrist, especially wrist extension (e.g. turning a screwdriver) and lifting movements.

Symptoms associated with tennis elbow include, but are not limited to, radiating pain from the outside of the elbow to the forearm and wrist, pain during extension of wrist, weakness of the forearm, a painful grip while shaking hands or torquing a doorknob, and not being able to hold relatively heavy items in the hand. The pain is similar to the condition known as *golfer's elbow*, but the latter occurs at the medial side of the elbow.

Causes

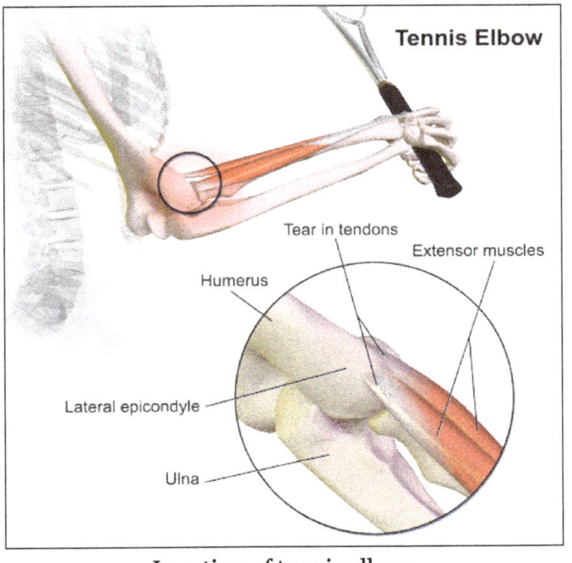

Location of tennis elbow.

Tennis elbow is a type of repetitive strain injury resulting from tendon overuse and failed healing of the tendon. In addition, the extensor carpi radialis brevis muscle plays a key role.

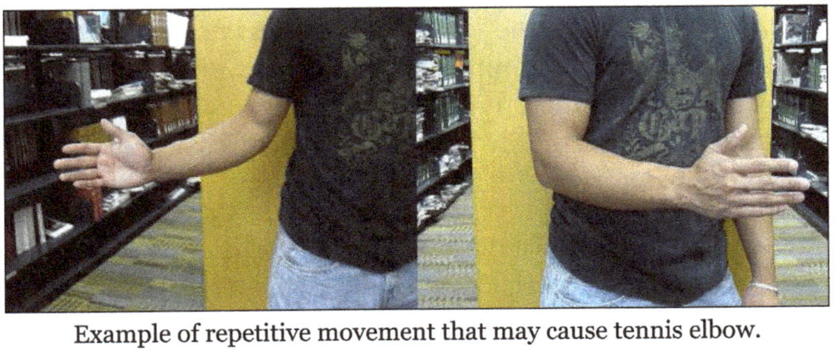

Example of repetitive movement that may cause tennis elbow.

Early experiments suggested that tennis elbow was primarily caused by overexertion. However, studies show that trauma such as direct blows to the epicondyle, a sudden forceful pull, or forceful extension cause more than half of these injuries. Repeatedly mis-hitting a tennis ball in the early stages of learning the sport causes shock to the elbow joint and may contribute to contracting the condition.

Pathophysiology

Histological findings include granulation tissue, microrupture, degenerative changes, and there is no traditional inflammation.

Longitudinal sonogram of the lateral elbow displays thickening and heterogeneity of the common extensor tendon that is consistent with tendinosis, as the ultrasound reveals calcifications, intrasubstance tears, and marked irregularity of the lateral epicondyle. Although the term "epicondylitis" is frequently used to describe this disorder, most histopathologic findings of studies have displayed no evidence of an acute, or a chronic inflammatory process. Histologic studies have demonstrated that this condition is the result of tendon degeneration, which replaces normal tissue with a disorganized arrangement of collagen. Therefore, the disorder is more appropriately referred to as *tendinosis* or *tendinopathy* rather than *tendinitis*.

Colour Doppler ultrasound reveals structural tendon changes, with vascularity and hypo-echoic areas that correspond to the areas of pain in the extensor origin.

The pathophysiology of lateral epicondylitis is degenerative. Non-inflammatory, chronic degenerative changes of the origin of the extensor carpi radialis brevis (ECRB) muscle are identified in surgical pathology specimens. It is unclear if the pathology is affected by prior injection of corticosteroid.

Tennis players generally believe tennis elbow is caused by the repetitive nature of hitting thousands of tennis balls, which leads to tiny tears in the forearm tendon attachment at the elbow.

The extensor digiti minimi also has a small origin site medial to the elbow that this condition can affect. The muscle involves the extension of the little finger and some extension of the wrist allowing for adaption to "snap" or flick the wrist—usually associated with a racquet swing. Most often, the extensor muscles become painful due to tendon breakdown from over-extension. Improper form or movement allows for power in a swing to rotate through and around the wrist—creating a moment on that joint instead of the elbow joint or rotator cuff. This moment causes pressure to build impact forces to act on the tendon causing irritation and inflammation.

At least one author questions that lateral epicondylitis is caused by repetitive micro-trauma/overuse, maintaining the theory is likely overstated and lacks scientific support.

Other speculative risk factors for lateral epicondylitis include taking up tennis later in life, unaccustomed strenuous activity, decreased mental chronometry and speed and repetitive eccentric contraction of muscle (controlled lengthening of a muscle group).

Prevention

Where lateral epicondylitis is caused by playing tennis, another factor of tennis elbow injury is experience and ability. The proportion of players who reported a history of tennis elbow had an increased number of playing years. As for ability, poor technique increases the chance for injury much like any sport. Therefore, an individual must learn proper technique for all aspects of their sport. The competitive level of the athlete also affects the incidence of tennis elbow. Class A and B players had a significantly higher rate of tennis elbow occurrence compared to class C and novice players. However, an opposite, but not statistically significant, trend is observed for the recurrence of previous cases, with an increasingly higher rate as ability level decreases.

Other ways to prevent tennis elbow:

- Decrease the amount of playing time if already injured or feeling pain in outside part of the elbow.
- Stay in overall good physical shape.
- Strengthen the muscles of the forearm: (pronator quadratus, pronator teres, and supinator muscle)—the upper arm: (biceps, triceps)—and the shoulder (deltoid muscle) and upper back (trapezius). Increased muscular strength increases stability of joints such as the elbow.
- Like other sports, use equipment appropriate to your ability, body size, and muscular strength.
- Avoid any repetitive lifting or pulling of heavy objects (especially over your head).

Vibration dampers (otherwise known as "gummies") are not believed to be a reliable preventative measure. Rather, proper weight distribution in the racket is thought to be a more viable option in negating shock.

Treatment

Evidence for the treatment of lateral epicondylitis before 2010 was poor. There were clinical trials addressing many proposed treatments, but the trials were of poor quality.

In some cases, severity of tennis elbow symptoms mend without any treatment, within six to 24 months. Tennis elbow left untreated can lead to chronic pain that degrades quality of daily living.

Physical Therapy

There are several recommendations regarding prevention, treatment, and avoidance of recurrence that are largely speculative including stretches and progressive strengthening exercises to prevent re-irritation of the tendon and other exercise measures.

One way to help treat minor cases of tennis elbow is simply to relax the affected arm. The rest lets stress and tightness within the forearm slowly relax and eventually have the arm in working condition—in a day or two, depending on the case.

Eccentric exercise using a rubber bar is highly effective at eliminating pain and increasing strength. The exercise involves grasping a rubber bar, twisting it, then slowly untwisting it. Although it can be considered an evidence-based practice, long-term results have not yet been determined.

There are differences in opinions on whether it is okay if pain occurs during these exercises. Some suggest pain of less than 5/10 is okay.

Moderate evidence exists demonstrating that joint manipulation directed at the elbow and wrist and spinal manipulation directed at the cervical and thoracic spinal regions results in clinical changes to pain and function. There is also moderate evidence for short-term and mid-term effectiveness of cervical and thoracic spine manipulation as an add-on therapy to concentric and eccentric stretching plus mobilisation of wrist and forearm. Although not yet conclusive, the short-term analgesic effect of manipulation techniques may allow more vigorous stretching and strengthening exercises, resulting in a better and faster recovery process of the affected tendon in lateral epicondylitis.

Low level laser therapy, administered at specific doses and wavelengths directly to the lateral elbow tendon insertions, may result in short-term pain relief and less disability.

Orthotic Devices

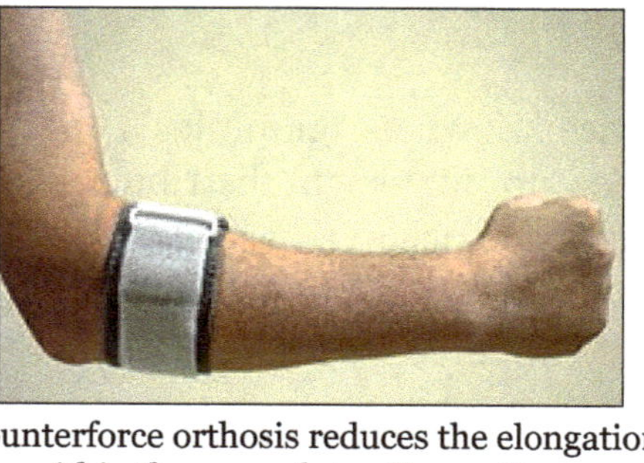

Counterforce orthosis reduces the elongation within the musculotendinous fibers.

Orthosis is a device externally used on the limb to improve the function or reduce the pain. Orthotics may be useful in tennis elbow, however long-term effects are unknown. There are two main types of orthoses prescribed for this problem: counterforce elbow orthoses and wrist extension orthoses.

Counterforce orthosis has a circumferential structure surrounding the arm. This orthosis usually has a strap which applies a binding force over the origin of the wrist extensors. The applied force by orthosis reduces the elongation within the musculotendinous fibers. Wrist extensor orthosis maintains the wrist in the slight extension. This position reduces the overloading strain at the lesion area.

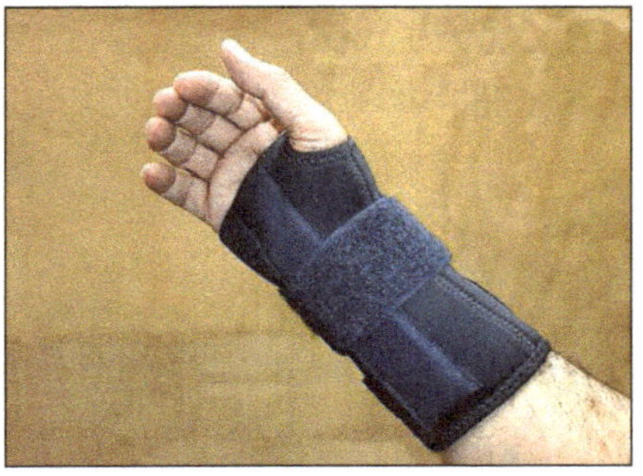

Wrist extensor orthosis reduces the overloading strain at the lesion area.

Studies indicated both type of orthoses improve the hand function and reduce the pain in people with tennis elbow. Extracorporeal shockwave therapy, while safe, is of unclear benefit.

Achilles Tendon Rupture

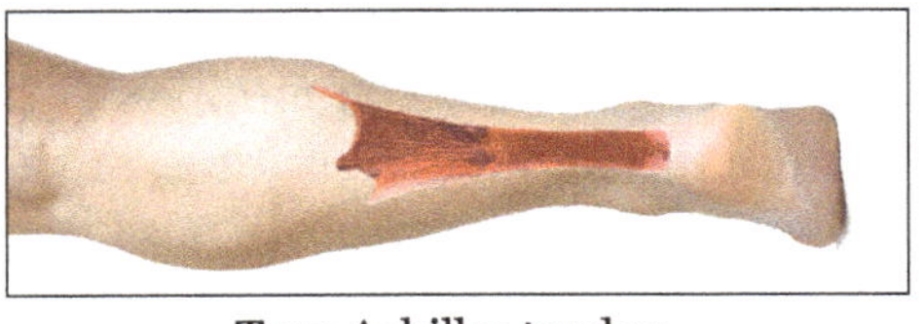

Torn Achilles tendon.

The Achilles tendon is the strongest and thickest tendon in the body. It attaches the calf muscles (soleus and gastrocnemius) to the heel bone (calcaneus). The tendon transmits force from the contracting calf muscles to the calcaneus to cause the foot action of plantar flexion (foot pointed down) that is important in walking, running, jumping and change of direction activities. Although the Achilles tendon is the strongest tendon in the body, it is also the tendon most commonly torn or ruptured.

The most common causes of rupture are:

- Sudden plantar flexion (foot moving downward) such as taking off to jump.
- Unplanned or forced dorsiflexion (foot moving upward) such as landing a jump or stepping into a hole.
- Direct trauma to the tendon. Most Achilles tendon ruptures occur in sports that require running, jumping and change of direction.

The typical age for rupture occurs between 30–40 years of age and is significantly more common in males than females. Older adults can also rupture the Achilles tendon and are more inclined to have degenerative partial tearing of the tendon. Other risk factors for Achilles tendon rupture include use of Fluoroquinolone antibiotics and direct steroid injections into the tendon.

The diagnosis of an Achilles tendon rupture is made from clinical history, physical exam and diagnostic testing. Most patients who sustain an Achilles tendon rupture report a pop and a feeling of being kicked or shot in the back of the leg. On exam, there is a palpable divot or gap in the area of the rupture along with significant swelling. Patients will demonstrate a positive Thompson test, performed by squeezing the calf muscle while the patient lies prone. This test is positive when the calf is squeezed and plantarflexion does not occur. Diagnostic testing such as an Ultrasound or MRI (magnetic resonance imaging) may be used to determine if there is a complete or partial tear.

Treatment options for an Achilles tendon rupture include surgical repair and conservative non-surgical rehabilitation. Decision making is based on age, past medical history and desired level of functional return. Conservative non-surgical treatment includes rehabilitation with initial immobilization followed by gentle range of motion and progressive strengthening to regain function. Most surgical procedures to repair a torn Achilles tendon include an open longitudinal incision medial to the Achilles tendon.

The incision is made medial to the tendon to improve skin healing and to reduce the risk of scarring to the underlying tendon repair. Once the incision is made and the rupture is identified, clamps are used to match the ends together in an optimal tendon length. A primary repair of the two ends of the tendon is performed by stitching them together. There are many different stitching techniques to repair the tendon. The type used will depend on the surgeon, the type of rupture, and tissue quality.

Sometimes the repair is augmented or strengthened using fascia or tendon. A gastrocnemius aponeurosis augmentation is performed when a 1–2 cm wide by 8 cm long flap is made and turned down over the repair and sutured to reinforce the repair. The area that the flap was harvested from is then stitched together. In cases of tendon degeneration, or tendiosis, this may help strengthen the repaired tendon.

Historically it has been thought that a surgically repaired Achilles tendon offered a significantly smaller risk of re-rupture rate and increased strength in comparison to non- surgical treatment. The major risks associated with surgery include infection, deep vein thrombosis (DVT) and difficulty with wound closure. Recent studies suggest similar rupture rates, strength and mobility between surgery and non-surgery approaches to the management of Achilles tendon ruptures. The best approach varies for each individual. Your surgeon and you will determine what is best for you by discussing your specific injury and goals.

Rehabilitation following Achilles tendon repair is vital in regaining motion, strength and function. Initially a walking boot is used for the first 4–5 weeks. Gradually more weight bearing and mobility is allowed to prevent stiffness post-operatively. The rehabilitation progresses slowly into strengthening, gait and balancing activities. Rehabilitation guidelines are presented in a criterion based progression. General time frames refer to the usual pace of rehabilitation. Individual patients will progress at different rates depending on their age, associated injuries, pre-injury health status, rehab compliance, tissue quality and injury severity. Specific time frames, restrictions and precautions may also be given to enhance wound healing and to protect the surgical repair/reconstruction.

Phase I: Surgery to 2 Weeks after Surgery

Appointments:

- Rehabilitation appointments begin 14-16 days after surgery.

Rehabilitation Goals:

- Protection of the surgically repaired tendon.
- Wound healing.

Precautions:

- Continuous use of the boot in locked plantarflexion (20-30°).
- Touchdown weight bearing (TDWB) using the axillary crutches.
- Keep the incision dry.
- Watch for signs of infection.
- Avoid long periods of dependent positioning of the foot during the first week to assist in wound healing.

Cardiovascular Exercise:

- Upper Body Ergometer (UBE) circuit training.

Progression Criteria:

- Two weeks after surgery.

Phase II: Begin after Meeting Phase 1 Criteria, usually 2 -4 Weeks after Surgery

Appointments:

- Rehabilitation appointments are 1-2 times per week.

Rehabilitation Goals:

- Normalize gait with weight bearing as tolerated (WBAT) using the boot and axillary crutches.
- Protection of the post-surgical repair.
- Active dorsiflexion to neutral.

Suggested Therapeutic Exercise:

- Ankle range of motion (ROM) with respect to precautions.
- Pain-free isometric ankle inversion, eversion, dorsiflexion and sub-max plantarflexion.
- Open chain hip and core strengthening.

Cardiovascular Exercise:

- Upper extremity circuit training or UBE.

Progression Criteria:

- Six weeks post-operatively.
- Pain-free active dorsiflexion to 0°.
- No wound complications.
- If wound complications occur, consult with a physician.

Phase III: Begin after Meeting Phase II Criteria, usually 6 to 8 Weeks after Surgery

Appointments:

- Rehabilitation appointments are once a week.

Rehabilitation Goals:

- Normalize gait on level surfaces without boot or heel lift.
- Single leg stand with good control for 10 seconds.
- Active ROM between 5° of dorsiflexion and 40° of plantarflexion.

Precautions:

- Slowly wean from use of the boot: Begin by using 1-2 ¼ inch heel lifts in tennis shoes for short distances on level surfaces then gradually remove the heel lifts during the 5th and 8th week depending on the surgeon.

- Avoid over-stressing the repair (avoid large movements in the sagittal plane; any forceful plantarflexion while in a dorsiflexed position; aggressive passive ROM; and impact activities).

Suggested Therapeutic Exercise:

- Frontal and sagittal plane stepping drills (side step, cross-over step, grapevine step).
- Active ankle ROM.
- Gentle gastroc/soleus stretching.
- Static balance exercises (begin in 2 foot stand, then 2 foot stand on balance board or narrow base of support and gradually progress to single leg stand).
- 2 foot standing nose touches.
- Ankle strengthening with resistive tubing.
- Low velocity and partial ROM for functional movements (squat, step back, lunge).
- Hip and core strengthening.
- Pool exercises if the wound is completely healed.

Cardiovascular Exercise:

Upper extremity circuit training or UBE.

Progression Criteria:

- Normal gait mechanics without the boot.
- Squat to 30° knee flexion without weight shift.
- Single leg stand with good control for 10 seconds.
- Active ROM between 5° of dorsiflexion and 40° of plantarflexion.

Phase IV: Begin after Meeting Phase III Criteria, usually 8 Weeks after Surgery

Appointments:

- Rehabilitation appointments are once every 1 - 2 weeks.

Rehabilitation Goals:

- Normalize gait on all surfaces without boot or heel lift.

- Single leg stand with good control for 10 seconds.
- Active ROM between 15° of dorsiflexion and 50° of plantarflexion.
- Good control and no pain with functional movements, including step up/down, squat and lunges.

Precautions:

- Avoid forceful impact activities.
- Do not perform exercises that create movement compensations.

Suggested Therapeutic Exercise:

- Frontal and transverse plane agility drills (progress from low velocity to high, then gradually adding in sagittal plane drills).
- Active ankle ROM.
- Gastroc/soleus stretching.
- Multi-plane proprioceptive exercises – single leg stand.
- 1 foot standing nose touches.
- Ankle strengthening – concentric and eccentric gastroc strengthening.
- Functional movements (squat, step back, lunge).
- Hip and core strengthening.

Cardiovascular Exercise:

- Stationary bike, Stair Master, swimming.

Progression Criteria:

- Normal gait mechanics without the boot on all surfaces.
- Squat and lunge to 70° knee flexion without weight shift.
- Single leg stand with good control for 10 seconds.
- Active ROM between 15° of dorsiflexion and 50° of plantarflexion.

Phase V: Begin after Meeting Phase IV Criteria usually 4 Months after Surgery

Appointments:

- Rehabilitation appointments are once every 1-2 weeks.

Rehabilitation Goals:

- Good control and no pain with sport/work specific movements, including impact.

Precautions:

- Post-activity soreness should resolve within 24 hours.
- Avoid post-activity swelling.
- Avoid running with a limp.

Suggested Therapeutic Exercise:

- Impact control exercises beginning 2 feet to 2 feet, progressing from 1 foot to other and then 1 foot to same foot.
- Movement control exercise beginning with low velocity, single plane activities and progressing to higher velocity, multi-plane activities.
- Sport/work specific balance and proprioceptive drills.
- Hip and core strengthening.
- Stretching for patient specific muscle imbalances.

Cardiovascular Exercise:

- Replicate sport/work specific energy demands.

Progression Criteria:

- Dynamic neuromuscular control with multi-plane activities, without pain or swelling.

Patellar Tendinitis

Patellar tendinitis, also known as jumper's knee, is an overuse injury of the tendon that straightens the knee. Symptoms include pain in the front of the knee. Typically the pain and tenderness is at the lower part of the kneecap, though the upper part may also be affected. Generally there is not pain when the person is at rest. Complications may include patellar tendon rupture.

Risk factors include being involved in athletics and being overweight. It is particularly common in athletes who are involved in jumping sports such as basketball and volleyball. The underlying mechanism involves small tears in the tendon connecting the kneecap with the shinbone. Diagnosis is generally based on symptoms and examination. Other conditions that can appear similar include infrapatellar bursitis, chondromalacia patella and patellofemoral syndrome.

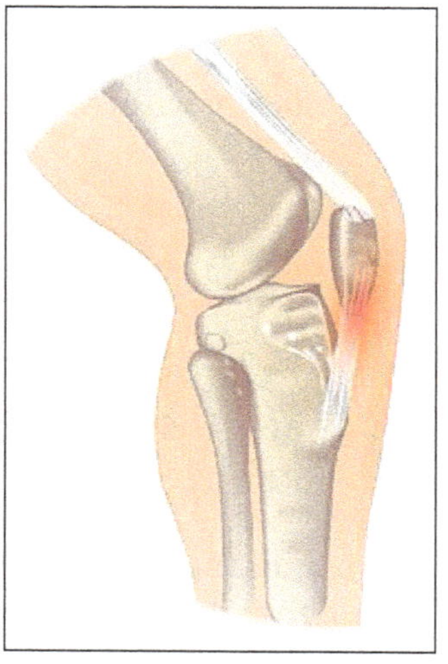

Location of the pain in patellar tendinitis.

Treatment often involves resting the knee and physical therapy. Evidence for treatments, including rest, however is poor. Recovery can take a year. It is relatively common with about 14% of athletes currently affected. Males are more commonly affected than females.

Treatment has two objectives: to reduce the inflammation and to allow the tendon to heal. When the knee is painful and swollen, you must rest it. Avoid stair climbing and jumping sports. Keep your knee straight while sitting, and avoid squatting. Let pain be your guide. You are aggravating the condition if you continue activities while experiencing pain. Mild discomfort or ache is not a problem but definite pain is a cause for concern. Ice your knee for 20 minutes, two or three times a day and after any sporting activities apply a bag of crushed ice over a towel. This reduces swelling, inflammation and pain. Aspirin, Aleve or Advil sometimes helps to relieve pain and reduce inflammation. A physical therapist or the doctor can recommend exercises to strengthen the muscles. Exercises can also be used to stretch and balance the thigh muscles. In some cases surgery may be indicated.

Chondromalacia Patella

The best treatment for patellofemoral syndrome is to avoid activities that compress the patella against the femur with force. This means avoiding going up and down stairs and hills, deep knee bends, kneeling, step-aerobics and high impact aerobics. Do not wear high heeled shoes. Do not do exercises sitting on the edge of a table lifting leg weights (knee extension).

An elastic knee support that has a central opening cut out for the kneecap sometimes helps. Applying ice packs for 20 minutes after exercising helps. Aspirin, Aleve or Advil sometimes helps.

Sports

Use your judgement. When your knees hurt, avoid sports that may aggravate your knee problems. Total rest may be required. When your knee is better after treatment, you should be able to enjoy many sports:

- Sports that aggravate patellar tendinitis and chondromalacia patella: Volleyball, basketball, soccer, distance running, racquetball, squash, football, weight-lifting (squats).
- Sports that may or may not cause symptoms: Cycling (it is best to keep the seat high and avoid hills), baseball, hockey, skiing and tennis.
- Sports that are easiest on the knees: Swimming (especially with a flutter kick), walking (avoid up and down hills), and cross-country skiing.
- Sports that are easiest on the knees: Swimming (especially with a flutter kick), walking (avoid up and down hills), and cross-country skiing.

Do not do the following exercises:

- Lunges.
- Squats.
- Stair-stepper machines.
- Leg extension machine.

The following exercises are OK to do if they cause no pain, grinding or swelling:

- Straight-leg lifting exercise.
- Stationary cycle (seat high, resistance low).
- Leg press (do not let the kneesbend past 90 degrees).
- Hamstring curl machine.

The following exercise program should be followed as instructed by the doctor or physical therapist. For the straight leg lift and short arc lift, ankle weights can be added to increase resistance and strength of the quadriceps. Generally, after 1 to 2 weeks, ankle weights can be added (starting at 1 pound) and increased by 1 pound per week until you build to 5 pounds. The exercises should be done daily until ankle weights are added. At this time, the straight-leg lift, short-arc lift and wall slides should be done every other day and the stretchesshould continue daily. When you have built up to 5 pounds on the straight-leg and short-arc lifts, continue the exercises 2 times per week for maintenance.

Straight Leg Lift

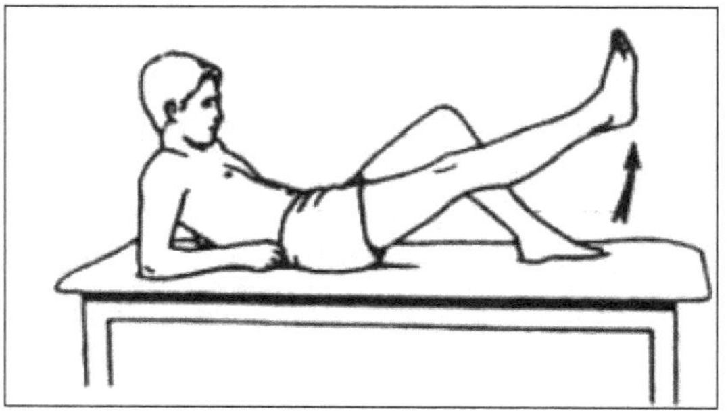

Tighten the quadriceps muscle so that the knee is flat, straight and fully extended- Try to raise the entire operated limb up off of the floor or bed. If you are able to keep the knee straight raise the limb to about 45 degrees, pause one second and then lower slowly to the bed. Relax and repeat. If the knee bends when you attempt to lift the limb off of t h e w, do not do this exercise. Keep trying to do the quadriceps setting exercise until you can lift the limb without letting the knee bend. Repeat 20 times.

Short Arc Lift

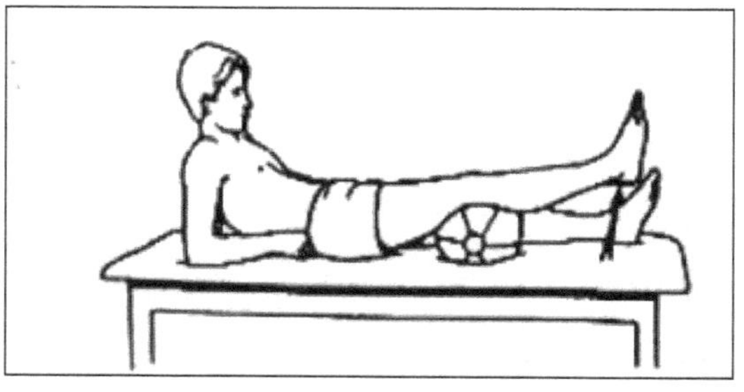

With the knee bent over a rolled up towel or blanket, lift the foot so that the knee fully straightens. Hold the knee locked in extension for 15 seconds, then slowly lower. Repeat 20 times.

Wall Slides

Stand upright with your back and buttocks touching a wall. Place the feet about 12 inches apart and about 6 inches from the wall. Slowly lower your hips by bending the knees and slide down the wall until the knees are flexed about 45 degrees. Pause five seconds and then slowly slide back up to the upright starting position. Doing this exercise too fast or too deep can aggravate your pain. Do not do this exercise if there is crunching or cracking at the kneecap or if it is painful. Do 3 sets of 10 to 15 repetitions.

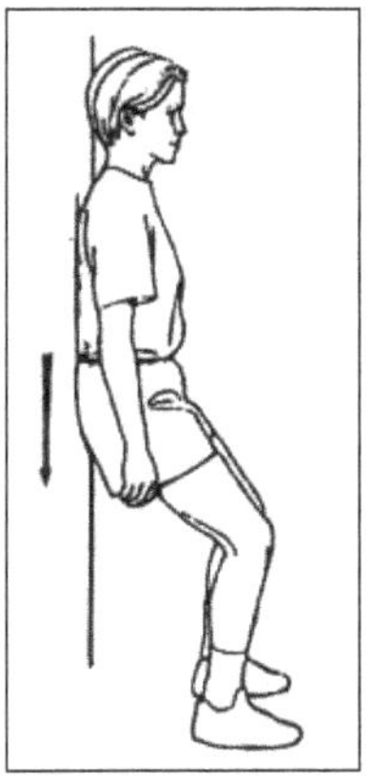

Hamstring Stretch

Perform this stretch in the position illustrated at the right. Bend slowly forward at the hips, keeping the knee fully extended until you feel gentle stretch in the back of your thigh and knee. Hold the stretch for 15 to 20 seconds and repeat 3 to 5 times.

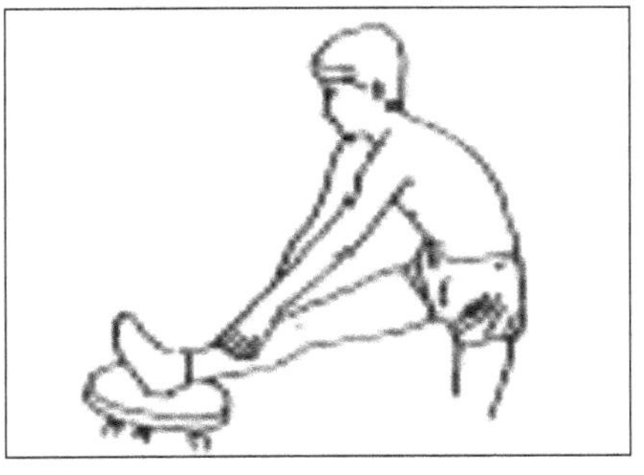

Quadriceps Stretch

This stretch is performed in the position illustrated at the right. Lean gently backward as if bringing you heel toward the buttock. When a stretch is felt in the front of the thigh and knee, hold 15 to 20 seconds for 3 to 5 repetitions.

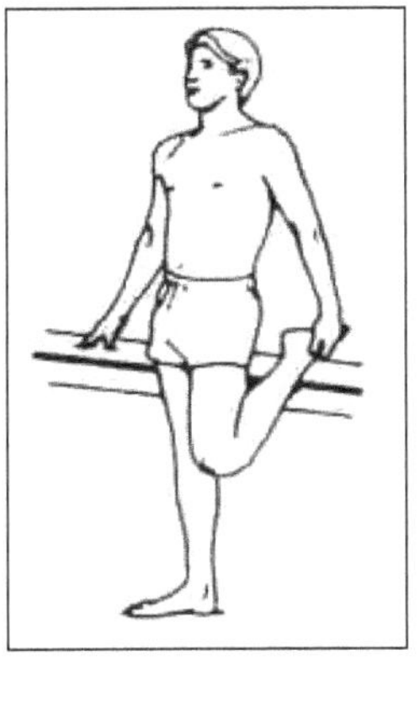

Calf Stretch

In the position illustrated, keep the heel flat on the floor and the knee fully extended. Lean forward at the hips with the arms supporting your weight. When you feel a gentle stretch in the back of your calf and knee, hold for 15 to 20 seconds, 3 to 5 repetitions.

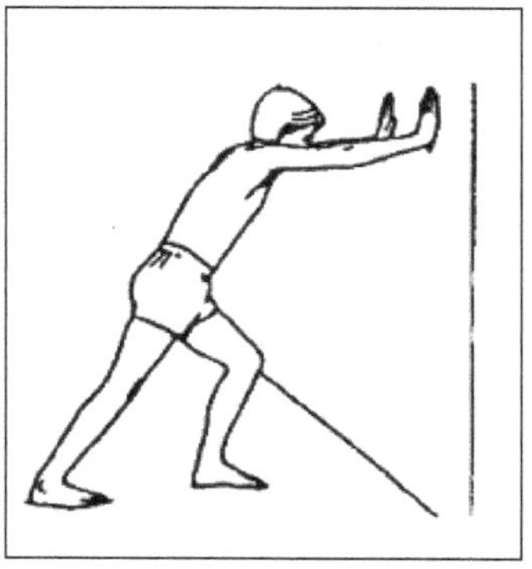

Lateral Hip and Thigh Stretch

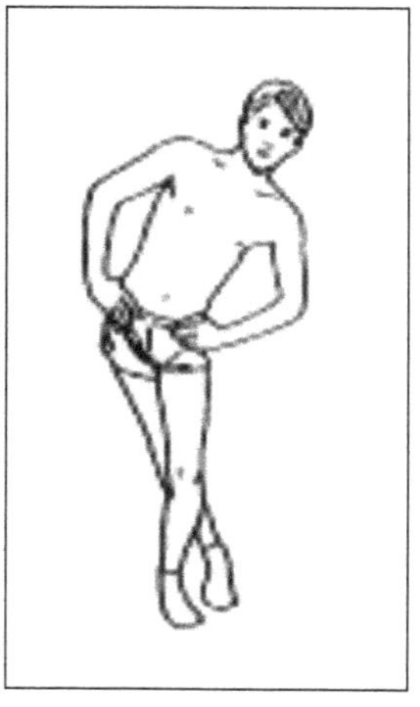

Cross your left (right) leg over in front of the other. Lean to the left (right), bending at the waist and letting your right (left) hip jut out. When you feel a gentle stretch in the out side of hip, hold 15 to 20 seconds,3 to 5 repetitions.

Patellar Dislocation

A patellar dislocation is a knee injury in which the patella (kneecap) slips out of its normal position. Often the knee is partly bent, painful and swollen. The patella is also often felt and seen out of place. Complications may include a patella fracture or arthritis.

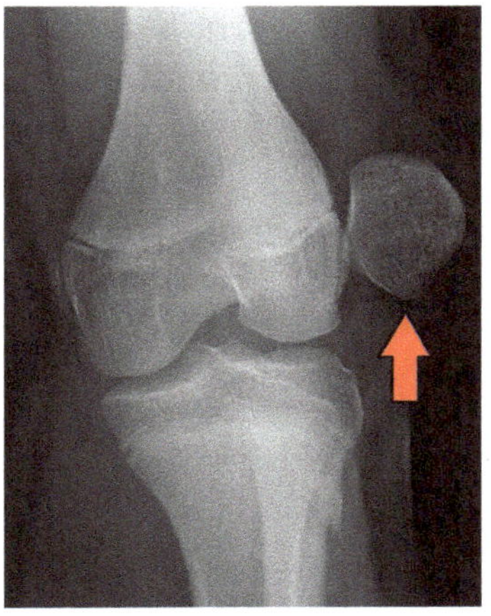

X-ray showing a patellar dislocation, with the patella out to the side.

A patellar dislocation typically occurs when the knee is straight and the lower leg is bent outwards when twisting. Occasionally it occurs when the knee is bent and the patella is hit. Commonly associated sports include soccer, gymnastics, and ice hockey. Dislocations nearly always occur away from the midline. Diagnosis is typically based on symptoms and supported by X-rays.

Reduction is generally done by pushing the patella towards the midline while straightening the knee. After reduction the leg is generally splinted in a straight position for a few weeks. This is then followed by physical therapy. Surgery after a first dislocation is generally of unclear benefit. Surgery may be indicated in those who have broken off a piece of bone within the joint or in which the patella has dislocated multiple times.

Patellar dislocations occur in about 6 per 100,000 people per year. They make up about 2% of knee injuries. It is most common in those 10 to 17 years old. Rates in males and females are similar. Recurrence after an initial dislocation occurs in about 30% of people.

Signs and Symptoms

People often describe pain as being “inside the knee cap.” The leg tends to flex even when relaxed. In some cases, the injured ligaments involved in patellar dislocation do not allow the leg to flex almost at all.

Risk Factors

A predisposing factor is tightness in the tensor fasciae latae muscle and iliotibial tract in combination with a quadriceps imbalance between the vastus lateralis and vastus medialis muscles can play a large role, found, mainly, in women with higher level the physical activity. Moreover, women with patellofemoral pain may show increased Q-angle compared with women without patellofemoral pain.

Another cause of patellar symptoms is *lateral patellar compression syndrome*, which can be caused from lack of balance or inflammation in the joints. The pathophysiology of the kneecap is complex, and deals with the osseous soft tissue or abnormalities within the patellofemoral groove. The patellar symptoms cause knee extensor dysplasia, and sensitive small variations affect the muscular mechanism that controls the joint movements.

24% of people whose patellas have dislocated have relatives who have experienced patellar dislocations.

Athletic Population

Patellar dislocation occurs in sports that involve rotating the knee. Direct trauma to the knee can knock the patella out of joint.

Anatomical Factors

People who have larger Q angles tend to be more prone to having knee injuries such as dislocations, due to the central line of pull found in the quadriceps muscles that run from the anterior superior iliac spine to the center of the patella. The range of a normal Q angle for men ranges from <15 degrees and for females <20 degrees, putting females at a higher risk for this injury. An angle greater than 25 degrees between the patellar tendon and quadriceps muscle can predispose a person to patellar dislocation.

In patella alta, the patella sits higher on the knee than normal. Normal function of the VMO muscle stabilizes the patella. Decreased VMO function results in instability of the patella.

Forces

When there is too much tension on the patella, the ligaments will weaken and be susceptible to tearing ligaments or tendons due to shear force or torsion force, which then displaces the kneecap from its origination. Another cause that patellar dislocation can occur is when the trochlear groove that has been completely flattened is defined as trochlear dysplasia. Not having a groove because the trochlear bone has flattened out can cause the patella to slide because nothing is holding the patella in place.

Mechanism of Injury

Patellar dislocations occur by:

- A direct impact that knocks the patella out of joint.
- A twisting motion of the knee, or ankle.
- A sudden lateral cut.

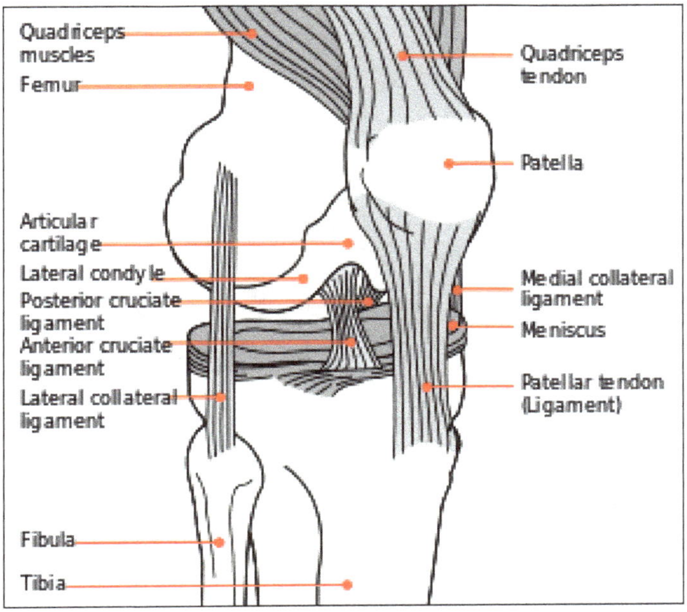

Anatomy of the Knee.

Anatomy of the Knee

The patella is a triangular sesamoid bone which is embedded in tendon. It rests in the patellofemoral groove, an articular cartilage-lined hollow at the end of the thigh bone (femur) where the thigh bone meets the shin bone (tibia). Several ligaments and tendons hold the patella in place and allow it to move up and down the patellofemoral groove when the leg bends. The top of the patella attaches to the quadriceps muscle via the quadriceps tendon, the middle to the vastus medialis obliquus and vastus lateralis muscles, and the bottom to the head of the tibia (tibial tuberosity) via the patellar tendon, which is a continuation of the quadriceps femoris tendon. The medial patellofemoral ligament attaches horizontally in the inner knee to the adductor magnus tendon and is the structure most often damaged during a patellar dislocation. Finally, the lateral collateral ligament and the medial collateral ligament stabilize the patella on either side. Any of these structures can sustain damage during a patellar dislocation.

Treatment

Two types of treatment options are typically available:

- Surgery.
- Conservative treatment (rehabilitation and physical therapy).

Surgery may impede normal growth of structures in the knee, so doctors generally do not recommend knee operations for young people who are still growing. There are also risks of complications, such as an adverse reaction to anesthesia or an infection.

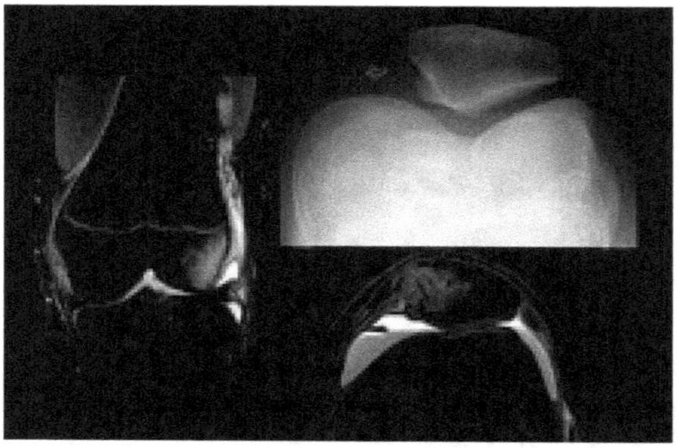

X-ray and MRI after luxation of the patella. There is a fragment and bone bruise at the medial surface of the patella and in the corresponding surface of the lateral condyle of the femur. The medial retinaculum of the patella is disrupted.

When designing a rehabilitation program, clinicians consider associated injuries such as chipped bones or soft tissue tears. Clinicians take into account the person's age, activity level, and time needed to return to work and/or athletics. Doctors generally only recommend surgery when other structures in the knee have sustained severe damage, or specifically when there is:

- Concurrent osteochondral injury.
- Continued gross instability.
- Palpable disruption of the medial patellofemoral ligament and the vastus medialis obliquus.
- High-level athletic demands coupled with mechanical risk factors and an initial injury mechanism not related to contact.

Supplements like glucosamine and NSAIDs can be used to minimize bothersome symptoms.

Rehabilitation

An effective rehabilitation program reduces the chances of re-injury and of other knee-related problems such as patellofemoral pain syndrome and osteoarthritis. Most patella dislocations are initially immobilized for the first 2–3 weeks to allow the stretched structures to heal. Rehabilitation focuses on maintaining strength and range of motion to reduce pain and maintain the health of the muscles and tissues around the knee joint. The objective to any good rehabilitation program is to reduce pain, swelling and stiffness as well as increase range of motion. A common rehabilitation plan is to strengthen both the hip abductors, hip external rotators and the quadricep muscles. Commonly used exercises include isometric quadricep sets, side lying clamshells, leg dips with internal tibial rotation, etc. The idea is that because the medial side is most often stretched by the more common lateral dislocation, medial strengthening will add more stabilizing support. With progression more intense range of motion exercises are incorporated.

Climbing Injuries

Climbers sustain a variety of unique injuries related to specific activities and anatomical region. In the upper extremities, overuse injuries predominate with repetitive strain patterns from training.

Like many athletes, climbers often experience rotator cuff tendonitis, impingement, and tears. Other common shoulder injuries seen in climbers include rupture of the long head of the biceps, SLAP lesions, AC sprains, glenohumeral dislocation, and muscular strains of the latissimus dorsi, rhomboid, and lower trapezius.

Specialized holds and maneuvers in sport climbing biomechanically affect the forearm and elbow. As an example, improper form often coupled with overuse can lead to injury such as climber's elbow. Climber's elbow, which represents a strain of the brachialis, distal biceps strain or tear, and posterior interosseous nerve compression, can cause anterior elbow pain. Overuse from grips can predispose climbers to medial epicondylitis. Other common injury patterns related to the forearm and elbow include strain or tear of the pronator teres, ulnar nerve compression, radio-capitellar compression, extensor strain causing lateral epicondylitis, and triceps tendonitis.

The wrist and hand experience overuse related to holds. Many types of tendonitis/tenosynovitis patterns may be seen in the wrist (most commonly flexor carpi ulnaris), along with sprains from falls while wedged in a crack, retinacular injury, or triangular fibrocartilage complex injury. Carpal tunnel syndrome is more likely to occur in climbers, secondary to flexor tendon hypertrophy and edema. Climber's finger, or flexor pulley injury, commonly afflicts sport climbers and boulderers. Forces on the small joints of the fingers can cause effusions, synovial irritation and cartilage damage, resulting in "sausage fingers" seen in sport climbers. Tendonitis of the flexor digitorum superficialis (FDS) and flexor digitorum profundus (FDP) can be seen, as well as strain, tear, or laceration in climbers. Mechanical stress inherent in the biomechanics of individual grips (proper and improper) contributes to the development of FDS and FDP tendonitis and tendonosis. Tendonosis can progress to tenoperiostitis (progression of tendonosis involving periosteum). Falls and side strain can cause collateral ligament injury of the fingers. Climbers also can experience flexion contracture, stress fracture, epiphyseal fracture in young climbers, trigger fingers, Dupuytren's contracture, ganglion cysts, mallet fingers, or lumbrical tear/shift.

Specific hand grips affect injury patterns in climbing. With an open grip, FDP strain is greater than that on FDS but is easier on joints, ligaments, and tendons. The crimp grip (with closed ring) places the majority of strain on FDS, DIP joints, and the volar plate. Pocket grips tend to strain FDP and collateral ligaments, whereas vertical grips focus strain on FDS. Pinch grips, finger locks, hand stacks, and finger/fist jams can cause overuse strain and torque injuries.

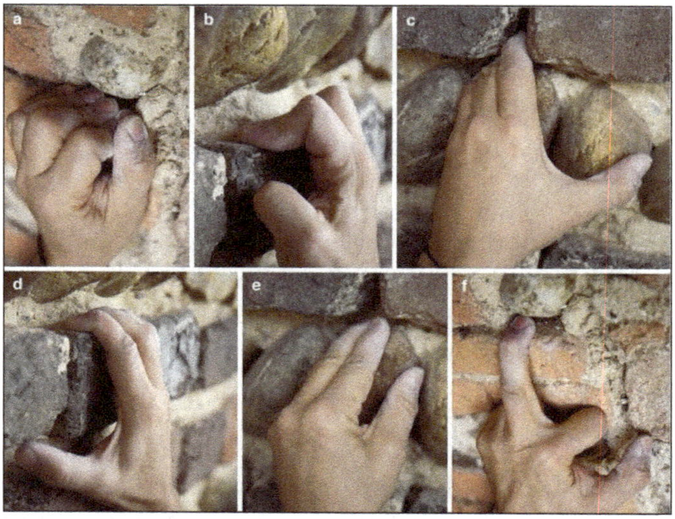

Crimp Grip, Open Grip, Pocket Grips, Vertical Grip (clockwise from upper left).

Most climbing injuries result from upper extremity overuse, but lower extremities also can be injured. With wide bridging between foot holds, climbers increase their risk for adductor strain or tear. Knee injury also can occur, but with a different mechanism in climbers. Meniscus tears can occur when routes require the climber to use a frog position with knee flexion and external rotation, applying an upward pushing force. ACL tears are typically related to a fall from bouldering height. Recent interest in the literature surrounds the lateral collateral ligamentous (LCL) complex and the heel-hook maneuver, described as a downward force placed on the heel with the hip flexed and externally rotated, knee flexed, and heel locked into a climbing hold, causing LCL complex strain.

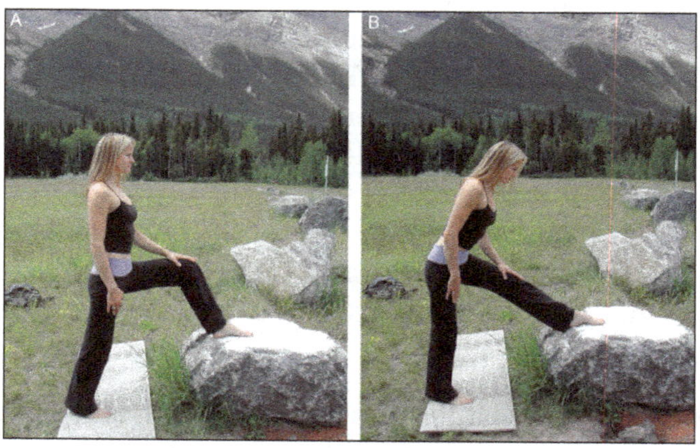

Heel hook, causing LCL complex stress.

Climbers also see various ankle and foot pathologies. Ankle sprains can occur as a consequence of climbing shoes tending to be small and preferring supination of the foot, leading to both dorsiflexion and the more common plantarflexion-inversion sprains. Climbers also may present with numbness or tingling secondary to shoe tightness. Falls from up to 3 m can predispose to ankle and foot trauma, but this risk can be reduced with adequate mats. Falls into a climbing surface or falls into ropes on an overhang may produce unique pathologies, which can produce osteochondritis dissecans (OCD) of the talus. The literature identifies posttraumatic OCD in climbers as a known complication of ankle sprain or dislocation. Other commonly seen pathologies include hallux valgus (common in those who climb >5 years), blisters, and toe nail contusion or loss.

As in many sports, core strength is critical to climbers, and climbing can impose specific injury patterns. The cervical spine is vulnerable to strains and degenerative changes, often exacerbated by belay position, the belayer vigilantly looking upward at the climber. Strains and disc injury involving the lumbar and thoracic spine can occur because of repeated stress from falls in harness causing hyperextension injury. Pectoralis imbalance can cause an increase in both thoracic kyphosis and lumbar lordosis. Climbers experience abdominal strains by reaching or during falls, particularly with an improperly fitted harness.

Lastly, injuries to the head and skin also are relatively common. Head injuries typically involve slamming into the rock with a fall or from falling rocks striking the climber, or more commonly, the belayer. Helmets protect both climbers and belayers when used. Falling rocks or pebbles and falling ropes also can lead to injuries of the eye. A flipped rope end can cause a hyphema to the anterior chamber of the eye, which can be prevented with eye protection. Abrasions, or "climber's rash," typically affect the lower extremities of less experienced climbers. Lacerations and sunburns occur with some regularity in outdoor climbers.

Climbing-specific Injuries

In general, climbing-specific injuries are less common than many other sport-related injuries. When injuries do occur in climbers, however, a lack in both scholarly literature and physician education regarding the clinical findings, diagnosis, and management of these injuries limits practitioners' ability to properly care for climbers in many circumstances. Understanding the conditions specific to climbing will help providers diagnose, treat, and communicate with their patients who climb. Mastering this interesting subset of injuries will broaden the provider's understanding of anatomy, biomechanics, and injury in general as well.

Climber's Finger

"Climber's finger" is an injury unique to climbers and generally represents some degree of strain or tear within the flexor pulley system in the digits of the hand. These injuries can either be acute or due to chronic overuse. Injury commonly involves A2,

A3, or A4 flexor pulleys, with injury to the A2 flexor pulley being the most common. Climber's finger has been shown to represent close to 30% of finger injuries seen in climbers. Different hand grips and specific techniques contribute to the development of pulley injuries. Roughly 50% of elite climbers have some degree of pulley injury. The mechanics of different grips place varying degrees of strain on the pulley system: at 90°, pulleys sustain more tension than the tendons themselves. The grading of the injury is based on the specific pulleys injured and the total number of pulleys affected.

	Grade 1	Grade 2	Grade 3	Grade 4
Injury	Pulley Strain	Complete rupture of A4 or partial rupture of A2 or A3.	Complete rupture of A2 or A3	Multiple rupture, such as A2/A3 and A2/A3/A4, or single rupture (A2 or A3 combined with lumbricails muscle or ligament damage
Therapy	Conservative	Conservative	Conservative	Surgical repair
Immobilization	None	10 d	10-14 d	Postoperative 14 d
Functional therapy	2-4 wk	2-4 wk	4 wk	4 wk
Pulley protection	Tape	Tape	Thermoplastic or soft-cast ring	Thermoplastic or soft-cast ring
Easy sport-specific activities	After 4 wk	After 4 wk	After 6-8 wk	4 months
Full sport-specific activities	6 wk	6-8 wk	3 months	6 months
Taping through climbing	3 months	3 months	6 months	>12 months

Climber's finger presents with a history of a "pop," swelling, and pain. Alternatively, climbers with a chronic-type injury present with a longstanding history of discomfort and feeling of relative weakness. Physical examination may demonstrate swelling and reproducible pain. Bowstringing of the flexor tendon of the affected digit also may be seen. The most commonly involved digit is the fourth digit of the nondominant hand. Musculoskeletal ultrasound (MSKUS) has been shown to be highly effective in diagnosing pulley ruptures with 98% sensitivity and 100% specificity; however, MSKUS is user dependent. Magnetic resonance imaging (MRI) will show edema and increased tendon-to-bone distance secondary to anterior subluxation of flexor tendons.

Treatment of climber's finger depends on the grade, with nonsurgical treatment preferred up to grade 3 injuries. With a grade 1 injury (pulley strain), immobilization is not recommended. Patients should undergo physical therapy (PT) for 2 to 4 wk, then return to light climbing at 4 wk. Full climbing can be resumed at 6 wk, with taping for stability for 3 months. Grade 2 injury (complete rupture of the A4 pulley or partial rupture of A2/A3) is best treated with 10 d of immobilization, followed by 2 to 4 wk of focused PT, with resumption of light climbing at 4 wk and full climbing at 6 to 8 wk. Again, taping for 3 months is recommended. With a grade 3 injury (complete A2 or A3 rupture), 10 to 14 d of immobilization is recommended. PT is scheduled for 4 wk, and the use of a tool such as a thermoplast also is suggested. These patients can return to light climbing at 6 to 8 wk and full climbing at 3 months, with taping for a total of 6 months. In all cases, nonsteroidal anti-inflammatory drugs (NSAID) are the only pharmacologic recommendation for control of pain and inflammation. Evidence is lacking, but platelet-rich plasma may be beneficial in treating lower grade pulley injuries.

In the case of a grade 4 injury (multiple pulley ruptures or A2/A3 rupture with lumbrical or ligament injury), surgery is indicated. The goal of surgery is to prevent flexion contractures and decreased range of motion secondary to flexor tendon bowstringing. Most recent studies have shown that pulley reconstruction versus repair has demonstrated superior postsurgical outcomes. The Widstrom technique (loop and a half) is most commonly used, but the Weilby repair is an alternative. Postoperatively, patients are immobilized for 14 d, followed by 4 wk of PT. Again, a thermoplast or ring is used. Patients return to light climbing in 4 months and progress to full climbing in 6 months, with taping for at least 1 year.

Prognosis is generally good for these injuries, and most climbers do well with conservative management. Approximately 10% of injuries lead to chronic or persistent pain. In general, surgical treatment should be considered when pain persists or with inability to return to prior climbing level.

Climber's Elbow

"Climber's elbow," a brachialis strain or tear at the musculotendinous junction, is another unique injury to climbers. Traversing climbs, engaging strong flexion and pronation of the elbow, with insufficient firing of biceps brachii in a flexed and pronated position, lead to compensatory firing of brachialis and acute or chronic overuse.

Climbers complain of pain with flexion and pronation, often presenting after a prolonged or difficult climb or after increased climbing intensity without sufficient rest between climbs. Physical examination often yields pain in the anterior elbow along the margin of the brachialis distally and is worsened with elbow flexion and pronation. Partial tears or ruptures present with swelling and ecchymosis.

Diagnosis is often made with physical examination and history, and MSKUS or MRI can be helpful in determining the degree of injury or in diagnosing elusive cases.

As with climber's finger, treatment of climber's elbow is generally conservative. Rest for 2 to 4 wk in the case of a strain with resumption of modified climbing only after the patient is pain free works well in milder cases. Climbing should be two to three levels below normal, with reduction in both frequency and intensity. PT can be effective when performed by a therapist skilled with the injury, with a focus on strengthening opposing muscle groups. Medication is limited to oral NSAIDs for inflammation and pain.

In the case of complete rupture, surgery is indicated and preferably performed within 1 to 2 wk of the injury. Surgical management is considered also if conservative management fails. Postoperatively, patients are splinted at 90° for 7 d, followed by a hinged brace set at 45° initially with advancement to full range of motion by 8 wk. Patients may begin strength-building exercises 1 wk postoperatively with isometric, low-intensity exercises to triceps and shoulder musculature. By the second week postoperatively, patients may begin strengthening biceps and brachialis utilizing isometric, low-intensity forearm flexion in a neutral plane. This will progress to active range of motion exercises in a single plane by the third to fourth week for flexion, pronation, and supination. Progressive resistance training is initiated at 8 wk postoperatively, and light sport-specific training may resume at roughly 3 months. Full recovery is expected to take place after several months. The specific length of activity restriction is individualized, and it depends on both the severity of the initial injury and progression through the rehabilitation process.

Whether treated conservatively or surgically, injured climbers typically resume full climbing levels without pain with adequate rest, PT, and strength training.

Extensor Hood Syndrome

Thought to be derived from extensive use of the crimp position, another injury seen almost exclusively in climbers is the extensor hood syndrome (EHS). EHS consists of the constellation of arthritic changes affecting the tendinous sheaths of the fingers with resultant irritation and inflammation. Chronic injuries to the flexor tendons of the hand often accompany EHS, and these are seen typically after years of climbing and a string of overuse hand injuries. Chronic finger injuries in climbers predispose toward progressive arthritic changes with the formation of significant bone spurring. These bone spurs produce irritation to the extensor tendons of the hand and present as a tenosynovitis.

Patients with EHS tend to have an extensive climbing history, with an average of 19 years of climbing experience. These patients have a history of chronic flexor and extensor tendon injuries with evidence of small joint arthritic changes. Patients generally complain of dorsal-sided pain of PIP and DIP joints (in the extensor hood region). A clinical picture similar to that of osteoarthritis may be present, including symptoms such as morning joint stiffness. Physical examination often elicits a 3° to 5° extension deficit of PIP and DIP joints and may demonstrate tenderness to palpation dorsally along bone spurs.

Both MSKUS and plain radiography play a role in diagnosis. Ultrasound, under skilled use, can demonstrate edema or effusion around the affected extensor hood. There also may be notable change in the path of the extensor tendons secondary to arthritic changes (spurs) along the extensor tendon pathway. With x-ray, dorsal bone spurs in proximity to PIP and DIP joint margins may be visualized, but the severity of radiographic findings rarely correlates to subjective symptom severity.

Conservative management of EHS remains the mainstay; however, this injury is relatively unstudied, with therapeutic evidence lacking. Treatment includes reduction of stress/load on the involved joints and tendons. NSAIDs are recommended for pain and inflammation, and some patients find relief with anti-inflammatory hand baths. Climbers with EHS should modify climbing to two levels below normal. Consideration also should be given to injection of cortisone into the affected tendon sheath.

Prognosis with conservative management has been excellent, but further study is needed. The study of EHS shows that all 12 patients recovered completely from both symptomatic and performance standpoints within 3 to 4 wk of initiation of conservative therapy.

Posttraumatic OCD

A fairly rare injury more unique to climbers is posttraumatic OCD. Any athlete can experience posttraumatic OCD, but climbers may have a unique predisposition due to mechanisms of potential injuries. Climbers may sustain foot and ankle injuries by falling from a distance or from slamming into the climbing surface.

Posttraumatic OCD presents as a potential complication of sprain or fracture and can be easily missed, as radiographs often do not show the injury. If a climber complains of persistent ankle pain beyond 6 wk, additional imaging should be considered. Serial x-rays may reveal the injury, but if negative in the setting of high clinical suspicion, MRI is indicated to rule out OCD.

Treating Climbers

A few general "pearls" will guide physicians caring for climbers. First, climbers must be adequately prepared through tendon strengthening, including opposing muscle groups, and with work on flexibility to avoid strain. Low weight and high-repetition training can be helpful. Body weight exercises and using training boards to strengthen and harden digits in preparation for climbing can help. Taping, used by many climbers, can prevent pulley injuries. A novel method of "H-tape" produces added protection by dividing the tape into two strips with a bridge in the middle, with the bridge placed at the volar PIP, then the strips placed circumferentially on either side of the dorsal PIP.

Paramount to injury prevention, climbers must give themselves ample recovery time, especially after the gym with multiple climbs at high difficulty levels. Rest for 24 h must be given for recovery after training and rest for 48 h after climbing or a hard training session. Climbers also must understand that with aging, the recovery time will be longer. Further, in the setting of overuse and injury, rest times need to be lengthened significantly and medical attention sought when not improving or with more significant injury.

Proper rehabilitation can take from weeks to months, depending on the injury, and careful attention must be given to help climbers understand how to modify their climbing in order to progress without sustaining further injury or preventing full recovery. Rehabilitation involves stretches, range-of-motion exercises, modalities, and low-weight/high-repetition strengthening, with a crescendo transition from modified climbing to full activity. Antagonist strengthening will ensure a balanced, long-term recovery. Modifications in technique, such as grip changes, may be necessary with certain injuries. Formal therapy with therapists experienced in climbing injuries will prove invaluable.

Physicians need to understand surgical indications and when to recognize failed conservative therapy. Compliance to postoperative protocols and rehabilitation proves critical to the ultimate surgical success.

Helping climbers to understand risks and to be prepared will aid in injury prevention. Climbers should have proper instruction and climb with trusted climbers, meticulously learning and rehearsing use of anchors, knots, and equipment. They need to understand their abilities and limitations. By keeping logs, including falls on ropes, and dating equipment and adhering to detailed inspection and equipment care (including storage and protection), climbers ensure safety. They should always have a plan and leave an itinerary with others and be prepared with maps/GPS, a first-aid kit, and adequate food, water, and protection from the environment. Helmets and eye protection should be used, particularly for outdoor climbing.

Rehabilitation in Spinal Cord Injury

When treating a person with a spinal cord injury, repairing the damage created by injury is the ultimate goal. By using a variety of treatments, greater improvements are achieved, and, therefore, treatment should not be limited to one method. Furthermore, increasing activity will increase his/her chances of recovery.

Acute Recovery

The rehabilitation process following a spinal cord injury typically begins in the acute care setting. Occupational therapy plays an important role in the management of SCI. Recent studies emphasize the importance of early occupational therapy, started immediately after the client is stable. This process includes teaching of coping skills, and physical therapy. Physical therapists, occupational therapists, social workers, psychologists and other health care professionals typically work as a team under the coordination of a physiatrist to decide on goals with the patient and develop a plan of discharge that is appropriate for the patient's condition. In the first step, the focus is on support and prevention. Interventions aim to give the individual a sense of control over a situation in which the patient likely feels little independence.

As the patient becomes more stable, they may move to a rehabilitation facility or remain in the acute care setting. The patient begins to take more of an active role in their rehabilitation at this stage and works with the team to develop reasonable functional goals.

Respiration

In the acute phase physical and occupational therapists focus on the patient's respiratory status, prevention of indirect complications (such as pressure sores), maintaining range of motion, and keeping available musculature active.

Depending on the Neurological Level of Impairment (NLI), the muscles responsible for expanding the thorax, which facilitate inhalation, may be affected. If the NLI is such that it affects some of the ventilatory muscles, more emphasis will then be placed on the muscles with intact function. For example, the intercostal muscles receive their innervation from T1–T11, and if any are damaged, more emphasis will need to be placed on the unaffected muscles which are innervated from higher levels of the CNS. As SCI patients suffer from reduced total lung capacity and tidal volume it is pertinent that physical therapists teach SCI patients accessory breathing techniques (e.g. apical breathing, glossopharyngeal breathing, etc.) that typically are not taught to healthy individuals.

Functional Electrical Stimulation

Physical therapists can assist immobilized patients with effective cough techniques, secretion clearance, stretching of the thoracic wall, and suggest abdominal support belts when necessary. The amount of time a patient is immobilized may depend on the level of the spinal cord injury. Physical therapists work with the patient to prevent any complications that may arise due to this immobilization. Other complications that arise from immobilization include muscle atrophy and osteoporosis, especially to the lower limbs, increasing the risk of fractures to the femur and tibia. While passive weight bearing of paralyzed lower extremities appears to be ineffective, stressing the bones through muscular contractions initiated by functional electrical stimulation (FES) has yielded positive results in some cases. The intensity, frequency, and duration of stress to the bones appear to be important determinants of improved bone parameters. Generally, the frequency is effective with three or more weekly exercise sessions. Studies of duration suggest that several months to one or more years of FES are necessary.

Improving Locomotor Function

Improvement of locomotor function is one of the primary goals for people with a spinal cord injury. SCI treatments may focus on specific goals such as to restore walking or locomotion to an optimal level for the individual. The most effective way to restore locomotion is by complete repair, but techniques are not yet developed for regeneration. Treadmill training, over groundtraining, and functional electrical stimulation can all be used to improve walking or locomotor activity. These activities work if neurons of the central pattern generator (CPG) circuits, which generate rhythmic movements of the body, are still functioning. With inactivity, the neurons of CPG degenerate. Therefore, the above activities are important for keeping neurons active until regeneration activities are developed. Sufficient evidence is found to conclude *which* locomotor training strategy improves walking function most for people with spinal cord injury. This suggests that it is not the type of training used, but the goals and the routines that have the biggest impact. Applying spinal cord stimulation (transcutaneous or epidurally) during weight supported walking have been shown to improve locomotor output.

Post-discharge Rehabilitation Therapy

Though rehabilitation interventions are performed during the acute phase, recent literature suggests that 44% of the total hours spent on rehabilitation during the first year after spinal cord injury, occur after discharge from inpatient rehabilitation. Participants in this study received 56% of their total physical therapy hours and 52% of their total occupational therapy hours after discharge. This suggests that inpatient rehabilitation lengths of stay are reduced and that post-discharge therapy may replace some of the inpatient treatment.

Functional Independence

Whether patients are placed in inpatient rehabilitation or discharged, occupational therapists attempt to maximize functional independence at this stage. Depending on the level of the spinal cord injury, whatever sparing the patient has is optimized. Bed mobility, transfers, wheelchair mobility skills, and performing other activities of daily living (ADLs) are just a few of the interventions that occupational therapists can help the patient with. A major problem for spinal cord injury patients is restricted range of motion. Massage therapy has been used to aid in range of motion rehabilitation. Literature has shown that participants with spinal cord injuries that had massage therapy added into their rehabilitation had significant improvement observed by physical therapist in functional living activities and limb range of motion. This could be due to the decrease in H-Reflex amplitudes measured by EMG that is critical for the comfort of spinal cord injury patients for reducing cramps and spasms.

ADLs can be difficult for an individual with a spinal cord injury; however, through the rehabilitation process, individuals with SCI may be able to live independently in the community with or without full-time attendant care, depending on the level of their injury.

Further interventions focus on support and education for the individual and caregivers. This includes an evaluation of limb function to determine what the patient is capable of doing independently, and teaching the patient self-care skills. Independence in daily activities like eating, bowel and bladder management, and mobility is the goal, as obtaining competency in self-care tasks contributes significantly to an individual's sense of self-confidence and reduces the burden on caregivers. Quality of life issues such as sexual health and function after spinal cord injury are also addressed.

Assistive Devices

Assistive devices such as wheelchairs have a substantial effect on the quality of life of the patient, and careful selection is important. Teaching the patient how to transfer from different positions, such as from a wheelchair into bed, is an important part of therapy, and devices such as sliding transfer boards and grab bars can assist in these tasks. Individuals who are able to transfer independently from their wheelchair to the driver's seat using a sliding transfer board may be able to return to driving in an adapted vehicle. Complete independence with driving also requires the ability to load and unload one's wheelchair from the vehicle. In addition to acquiring skills such as wheelchair transfers, individuals with a spinal cord injury can greatly benefit from exercise reconditioning. In the majority of cases, spinal cord injury leaves the lower limbs either entirely paralyzed, or with insufficient strength, endurance, or motor control to support safe and effective physical training. Therefore, most exercise training employs the use of arm crank ergometry, wheelchair ergometry, and swimming. In one study, subjects with traumatic spinal cord injury participated in a progressive exercise training program, which involved arm ergometry and resistance training. Subjects in the exercise group experienced significant increases in strength for almost all muscle groups when compared to the control group. Exercisers also reported less stress, fewer depressive symptoms, greater satisfaction with physical functioning, less pain, and better quality of life. Physical therapists are able to provide a variety of exercise interventions, including, passive range of motion exercises, upper body wheeling (arm crank ergometry), functional electrical stimulation, and electrically stimulated resistance exercises all of which can improve arterial function in those living with SCI. Physical therapists can improve the quality of life of individuals with spinal cord injury by developing exercise programs that are tailored to meet individual patient needs. Adapted physical activity equipment can also be used to allow for sport participation: for example, sit-skiis can be used by individuals with a spinal cord injury for cross-country or downhill skiing.

The patient's living environment can also be modified to improve independence. For example, ramps or lifts can be added to a patient's home, and part of rehabilitation involves investigating options for returning to previous interests as well as developing new pursuits. Community participation is an important aspect in maintaining quality of life.

Gait Training

Body weight supported treadmill training is another intervention that physiotherapists may assist with. Body weight supported treadmill training has been researched in an attempt to prevent bone loss in the lower extremities in individuals with spinal cord injury. Research has shown that early weight-bearing after acute spinal cord injury by standing or treadmill walking (5 times weekly for 25 weeks) resulted in no loss or only moderate loss in trabecular bone compared with immobilized subjects who lost 7-9% of trabecular bone at the tibia. Gait training with body weight support, among patients with incomplete spinal cord injuries, has also recently been shown to be more effective than conventional physiotherapy for improving the spatial-temporal and kinematic gait parameters.

A combination of Body weight supported treadmill training (BWSTT) and robotic-assisted BWSTT is being implemented into some training programs. The benefits include: (1) assist in reproducing leg movements and optimizing gait pattern (speed, step length, amplitude); (2) training sessions can be prolonged and walking speed can be adjusted, increasing motor outcome; (3) provides consistency of movement, where manual interventions/cues by a trainer may be variable (although a trainer should analyze the gait pattern and outcome measures of the training and supervise training). It is important to note that the patient must be an active participant during the robotic movements and try to move with the robot. This type of training would be implemented during the beginning of rehabilitation and progressed to independent locomotion as improvements are made. However, robotic-assisted BWSTT is expensive and often not affordable by physiotherapy clinics. As an alternative, the development of non-motorized exoskeletons are currently being investigated for patients with incomplete SCI. The development of the exoskeleton locomotor device would provide an inexpensive alternative to the robotic devices. The exoskeleton may be used in areas that can not afford robotic devices, or, in areas that can not provide adequate physiotherapy care.

Restorative neurology offers a different paradigm of treating spinal cord injury by focusing on the residual remaining motor control and on the intrinsic function of the sub-lesional spinal cord segments.

Exertional Rhabdomyolysis

Exertional rhabdomyolysis is a relatively uncommon but potentially fatal condition affecting athletes that requires prompt recognition and appropriate management.

Overuse injuries are common in athletes and present a variety of challenges. For many athletes, the medical management and return-to-sport considerations of overuse injuries involve many variables including the goals of the athlete, medical staff, family, coach, and administration. Although exertional rhabdomyolysis (ER) is relatively rare, the consequences can be fatal, and therefore, appropriate treatment should be initiated to limit morbidity and mortality.

Pathophysiology

Exertional rhabdomyolysis is characterized by the breakdown and necrosis of striated skeletal muscle after engaging in physical activity. Although there are several different mechanisms that can lead to skeletal muscle cell damage and death, the common final pathway is an increase in intracellular free ionized calcium to a level much higher than normal in the cytoplasm and mitochondria. In rhabdomyolysis secondary to trauma, the increase in intracellular calcium is caused by direct injury and rupture of the cellular membrane. ER also has an overproduction of heat, resulting in increased intracellular calcium via depletion of adenosine triphosphate (ATP). The loss of ATP causes dysfunction of Na/K–ATPase and Ca^{2+}ATPase pumps, leading to an increase of intracellular calcium. This increase in intracellular calcium leads to the activation of proteases and production of reactive oxygen species, eventually culminating into the death of the skeletal muscle cells. Necrosis of skeletal muscle cells releases intracellular contents causing pain, swelling, and potential end organ damage in the athlete.

Diagnosis

Exertional rhabdomyolysis may be an extreme continuation of delayed-onset muscle soreness. Affected individuals typically complain of proportional pain, tenderness, weakness, and swelling in the muscles affected following athletic activity. Elevated CK levels 5 times the upper limit of normal with these symptoms are required for diagnosis.

Black football players with sickle cell trait are at a 37 times higher risk of exertional-related death when compared with their non–sickle cell trait counterparts. The cause of this increase in mortality is not completely understood. The depletion of ATP that occurs with ER and the sickling nature of red blood cells may deplete skeletal muscle of oxygen or may represent an autoimmune phenomenon.[7] Elevated levels of CK are normal after exercise in healthy, asymptomatic individuals, and blacks have higher baseline CK levels. In 499 military recruits, peak CK levels occurred at day 7 of initial basic training (mean, 1226 IU/L; range, 56-35,056 IU/L). Recruits did not develop clinically significant ER, but a CK range considering ethnicity should be considered.

A cumulative increase in resting serum CK was noted in 22 Division I football players over the course of a single season. The peak CK range was 119 to 2834 IU/L after the ninth game of the season. A study comparing athletes with nonathletes in Greece noted that athletes have a significantly higher baseline CK level. The range for diagnosis of rhabdomyolysis differs for each laboratory, but traditionally, it includes an increase of CK 5 to 10 times the upper limit of normal. Significantly elevated CK must be present for the diagnosis of ER but should be made in association with the presenting clinical syndrome of muscle weakness, swelling, pain, and occasionally, darkening of the urine to differentiate rhabdomyolysis from other causes. Elevated levels of myoglobin will occasionally lead to darkened urine (tea or cola colored), with positive blood findings on urinalysis without red blood cells. Rapid clearance of myoglobin from the urine makes it a less sensitive indicator for ER, and it should not be used as the sole objective diagnostic marker.

Severe consequences of this condition include disseminated intravascular coagulation, acute kidney failure, hyperkalemia, and cardiac dysrhythmias. Elevated levels of myoglobin in the serum do not necessarily predispose an athlete to renal failure. Of the deaths that occurred in athletes because of this condition, other factors, including recent illness and cardiac ischemia, were listed as potential causes as well. Prompt recognition of these symptoms is paramount.

Treatment

In mild cases, ER may go undiagnosed and could be managed on an outpatient basis with oral hydration and rest. For an athlete with severe symptoms (CK greater than 5 times the upper limit of normal or darkening of the urine), hospital admission is indicated for intravenous hydration with normal saline (1-2 L/h) maintaining a urine output of 200 mL/h. Along with intravenous hydration, the tracking of CK levels, kidney function, and electrolyte values is much easier to manage in an inpatient setting where continuous venovenous hemodialysis and other services are readily available. CK levels should be monitored daily. If levels continue to elevate past 48 to 72 hours from the time of injury, consultation of a nephrologist or surgeon should be considered, depending on the severity of kidney disease or presence of compartment syndrome. Continuous venovenous hemodialysis should be considered if the athlete is not be able to maintain appropriate volume or electrolyte balance. Diuretics (thiazides and loop diuretics) can further deteriorate kidney function in this setting and should be prohibited.

The initial rehabilitation program should be composed of exercise containing gradual resistive exercises to activate cell function and prevent energy deficiency. This would enable the exercise intensity of muscles to be placed below an aerobiosis. In general, the range of motion of joints should improve simultaneously. During the 1st stage of a rehabilitation program, manual efforts to secure a range of motions of joints may require some form of discomfort and perhaps some pain. Before recovering from complete joint mobilization, the 2nd stage of rehabilitation should increase gradually. The distal portion of the upper or lower part of the body should be manipulated gradually with very low intensity from 5 to 15 min using a non-weight bearing equipment. If no feeling of discomfort or pain is present within 24 h after the exercise, the 3rd stage of the rehabilitation program could be introduced. In the 3rd stage of the rehabilitation program, isotonic exercises such as stretching of the joints, modified flexion and extension of joints, or bench press should be gradually introduced. Modified flexion and extension of joints should start from forward tilted position with both hands touching the wall, and then proceed to a table, a footboard, or chairs, and finally to the floor to increase the joint mobility and exercise intensity. In the 4th stage of the rehabilitation program, one set of limited flexion and extension of the joints should be performed together with the normal exercise program. The limits of flexion and extension of joints is to restore performance capability before determination of RML without loss of range of motion of joints or pain.

Guidelines of O'Connor divide the rehabilitation program in 3 phases for athletes at low risk for RML. In Phase 1, CK and urinalysis are monitored during moderate resting. In Phase 2, the guidelines suggest the initiation of physical activity. In Phase 3, the guidelines suggest a gradual comeback to sports activity. They recommend 72 h of rest and ample water intake after the onset of RML in Phase 1. Eight hours of sleep has been recommended together with remaining in a heat-controlled environment in the presence of RML when accompanied with heat injury. Monitoring of CK and urinalysis every 72 h has also been recommended. Light physical activities in Phase 2 could be initiated after urinalysis results reveal CK levels below 5 times of the normal level. In cases where CK or the results of urinalysis are not normalized within 2 weeks, medical consultation was recommended. For Phase 2, physical activities considering self-paced distance should be practiced. The Phase 3 could be initiated along with necessary follow-ups when no clinical symptoms a represent during a 1-week follow-up in Phase 2. The rehabilitation program after the onset of RML should be advanced gradually while carefully monitoring symptoms.

Rotator Cuff Tendinitis

Rotator cuff tendinitis, or tendonitis, affects the tendons and muscles that help move your shoulder joint. If you have tendinitis, it means that your tendons are inflamed or irritated. Rotator cuff tendinitis is also called impingement syndrome.

This condition usually occurs over time. It can be the result of keeping your shoulder in one position for a while participating in activities that require lifting your arm over your head.

Athletes playing sports that require lifting their arm over their head commonly develop rotator cuff tendinitis. This is why the condition may also be referred to as:

- Swimmer's shoulder.
- Pitcher's shoulder.
- Tennis shoulder.

Sometimes rotator cuff tendinitis can occur without any known cause. Most people with rotator cuff tendinitis are able to regain full function of the shoulder without any pain.

Symptoms of Rotator Cuff Tendinitis

The symptoms of rotator cuff tendinitis tend to get worse over time. Initial symptoms may be relieved with rest, but the symptoms can later become constant. Symptoms that go past the elbow usually indicate another problem.

Symptoms of rotator cuff tendinitis include:

- Pain and swelling in the front of your shoulder and side of your arm.
- Pain triggered by raising or lowering your arm.
- A clicking sound when raising your arm.
- Stiffness.
- Pain that causes you to wake from sleep.
- Pain when reaching behind your back.
- A loss of mobility and strength in the affected arm.

Diagnosis

If you're having symptoms of rotator cuff tendinitis, your doctor will begin by examining your shoulder. You'll be checked to see where you're feeling pain and tenderness. Your doctor will also test your range of motion by asking you to move your arm in certain directions.

Your doctor may also test the strength of your shoulder joint by asking you to press against their hand. They may also examine your neck to check for conditions such as a pinched nerve or arthritis that can cause symptoms similar to rotator cuff tendinitis.

Your doctor may order imaging tests to confirm the diagnosis of rotator cuff tendinitis and rule out any other causes of your symptoms. An X-ray may be ordered to see if you have a bone spur. Your doctor may order an ultrasound or MRI scan to check for inflammation in your rotator cuff and signs of any tearing.

Treatment

Initial treatment of rotator cuff tendinitis involves managing pain and swelling to promote healing. This can be done by:

- Avoiding activities that cause pain.
- Applying cold packs to your shoulder three to four times per day.
- Taking nonsteroidal anti-inflammatory drugs (nsaids) like ibuprofen (advil) and naproxen (aleve).

Additional treatment may include:

Physical Therapy

Your doctor may refer you to a physical therapist. Physical therapy will initially consist of stretching and other passive exercises to help restore range of motion and ease pain.

Once the pain is under control, your physical therapist will teach you exercises to help regain strength in your arm and shoulder.

Steroid Injection

If your rotator cuff tendinitis isn't being managed by more conservative treatment, your doctor may recommend a steroid injection. This is injected into the tendon to reduce inflammation, which reduces pain.

Surgery

If nonsurgical treatment isn't successful, your doctor may recommend surgery. Most people experience full recovery after having rotator cuff surgery.

The most noninvasive form of shoulder surgery is accomplished via arthroscopy. This involves two or three small cuts around your shoulder, through which your doctor will insert various instruments. One of these instruments will have a camera, so your surgeon can view the damaged tissue through the small incisions.

Open shoulder surgery is usually not required for rotator cuff tendinitis. However, this method may be used if there are other problems in your shoulder, such as a large tendon tear.

Surgery involves recovery that consists of rest and physical therapy to restore strength and range of motion.

Post Operative Rehabilitation after Rotator Cuff Surgery

Immobilization versus Early Range of Motion

In addition to the surgical technique, a major contributor to successful outcomes after rotator cuff repair is the postoperative management. In general, rehabilitation protocols need to take into account the slow process of tendon healing to the bone. It has been shown with animal model that a tendon exposed to pressure and immobilization has better healing rates. Hatakeyama showed that there is less tension on the superior rotator cuff in 30° and 45° compared to 0° and 15° of abduction. Additionally, his group showed that the tension diminished if the humerus is in the scapular plane. Ghodadra-found factors that influence rehabilitation include the surgical approach, quality of the tendon, the localization and tear configuration as well as the etiology for the rupture (acute versus degenerative). Moreover, several studies have demonstrated that an open approach is associated with increased postoperative pain, which in turn leads to longer rehabilitation and lost time from work.

Despite the prolonged healing process of the tendon to bone, several authors advocate early mobilization with passive range of motion in order to overcome postoperative stiffness. These authors state that early motion does not have a negative effect on tendon healing. Keener in a randomized and prospective study evaluated 123 patients with either early passive ROM or delayed range of motion for 6 weeks. They reported no significant differences between the two groups in terms of tendon rate healing and also functional outcome. Thus the authors concluded that early ROM could be started in patients with small to medium sized tears under the age of 65 without any detriment to the postoperative healing and also functional outcome. In contrast to the above studies, Rokito and Severud looked at rehabilitation after open, mini-open and all-arthroscopic rotator cuff repairs, respectively. Both authors advocate immobilization for approximately 6 weeks with only little passive exercises. Severud showed a lower incidence of fibrous ankylosis after all-arthroscopic techniques with delay motion and stated the patient will return-tosports after six months. Regarding immobilization and its effect on range of motion, several authors reported postoperative stiffness with delayed motion for rotator cuff repairs is not a concern and that these patients will eventually regain their mobility and range of motion. Parsons showed in their retrospective cohort study that full-time sling immobilization without formal therapy for 6 weeks did not result in increased stiffness after one year.

Continuous Passive Motion

The role of continuous passive range of motion in rotator cuff repair patients is currently not clearly defined. Previous reports of CPM benefits have been extensively reported in total joint arthroplasty patients including decreased rates of knee manipulation, deep vein thrombosis and post-operative narcotics use, and resultant greater range of motion. Lastayo in a level I randomized controlled trial that compare the results of CPM to manual passive range of motions exercises after rotator cuff repairs and found no significant differences between the two groups in pain and disability (by SPADI), range of motion or isometric strength. However, the CPM group had less pain at 1 week post-operatively.

The benefits of continuous passive motion appear to be more significant when it is used in conjunction with traditional physical therapy. Studies have demonstrated significant short term improvement in terms of ROM with CPM plus PT, but the long term benefits of this combination were not found to be significant. Overall, studies suggest that CPM does have short term benefit in the improvement of ROM when it is prescribed with traditional physical therapy, but it lacks clear long term benefits and incurs higher overall cost.

Ice or Cryotherapy

Cryotherapy in total joint arthroplasty has demonstrated its benefits in terms of blood loss, postoperative pain, and range of motion, but the improvement is small and may not be of clinically significance. The role of cryotherapy in the immediate post-operative period has been well defined. Singh reported significant improvement in post-operative pain in continuous cryotherapy patients compared to control, which led to return to normal sleeping patterns and increased patient satisfaction. Physiologically, continuous cryotherapy decreases the temperatures in glenohumeral joint and subacromial space in the postoperative shoulder. This can potentially blunt the detrimental effects of proteolytics enzymes and improve overall pain control. Speer in a prospective study comparing post-operative patients fitted with cryotherapy to those that did not found cryotherapy resulted in less postoperative pain and perceived need for narcotics. Patients also had less swelling and pain during rehabilitation, resulting in improved rehabilitation effort.

Rotator Cuff Rehabilitation after Repair

Novel Modality for Rehabilitation

Aquatic rehabilitation: During the early phases shoulder rehabilitation, aquatic exercises can be utilized to complement land based AAROM in restoring glenohumeral range of motion as well as allow graduated resistance activities in a more protective and conducive environment. The beneficial properties of water have been utilized for centuries as a medium for rehabilitation, relaxation, and training as it offers many clinical advantages. The warmth and buoyancy of water enhance stretching, while the buoyancy also allows initiation of resistive exercise at a low and protective level that can be graduated up depending on the direction of movement. Furthermore, the water's viscosity provides enough resistance throughout a movement pattern in any plane . A warm-water pool provides an environment that may allow for increased soft tissue extensibility, as muscles may relax in a warm environment. Although a warm-water pool provides only superficial heat, temperature has been found to have a profound effect on the properties of collagen. Additionally, because buoyancy supports the arm and can make the activity passive, water makes certain movements easier to perform and optimal positions easier to maintain.

The pool is an ideal place to improve shoulder mobility, as the functional upward movement of the glenohumeral joint is assisted by buoyancy. As such, the patient may discover that normal movement patterns occur earlier in the pool than in a gravity environment. This movement is similar to active-assisted range of motion on dry land, but the buoyancy of the water now supports the recovering extremity. Buoyancy can be used in rehabilitation as assistance, support, or resistance depending on the direction of movement. Buoyancy-assisted exercise occurs when movements are in an upward direction, toward the surface of the water. These exercises are commonly used to increase mobility. Buoyancy-supported exercises are perpendicular to the upward thrust of buoyancy and parallel to the bottom of the pool. Typically, the limb floats just below the surface of the water. Examples of buoyancy-supported exercise include horizontal abduction and adduction of the shoulder with the patient standing upright. Buoyancy-resisted exercises are performed toward the bottom of the pool, directly opposing the upward thrust of buoyancy.

The reason for aquatic exercises being more protective is due both to the support of buoyancy and the negation of gravity. For example, horizontal abduction exercises in the pool do not require the same shoulder abductor work as the equivalent exercise on land. Golland found that exercises performed at 90° of abduction in the water were associated with significantly less electromyographic activity than land-based exercise.

Therefore aquatic therapy provides a supportive medium whereby protected active motion may begin at a much earlier stage in rehabilitation than land-based exercise, without compromising the repair integrity.

An important issue to note with aquatic exercise is the speed of movement. Although buoyancy-assisted, -supported, and -resisted activities seem intuitively obvious, the buoyancy component can be overridden by viscosity if the exercise occurs fast enough. For example, shoulder horizontal abduction and adduction is a buoyancy-supported exercise, and shoulder abduction is technically a buoyancy-assisted exercise, but these exercises can still be resistive if they are performed quickly enough to encounter resistance from the water's viscosity.

Other Novel Physical Therapy Modalities

Although commonly used to manage rotator cuff tear, the efficacy of physical therapy modalities such as transcutaneous electrical nerve stimulation, iontophoresis, and ultrasound in the postoperative setting remains controversial. There is a paucity of well-controlled clinical trials that have evaluated their role in patients with rotator cuff tear. These modalities may have an effect on pain and limited motion, but their impact on the underlying tear and repair is not known.

Different Phases of Therapy and Exercises

An ideal rehabilitation program is one that best allows for tendon to bone healing while preventing shoulder stiffness. However, because every patient and every rotator cuff tear is not often the same, it is important that any form of rehabilitation takes this difference into consideration for optimal results. For example, patients with large to massive rotator cuff tears are more likely to retear and therefore undergo a slower form of rehabilitation to protect the repair. Importantly, by delaying both motion to 6 weeks and strengthening to beyond 4 months, the conservative protocol allows Sharpey fibers to form at the tendon–bone junction before stressing the repair with resistive exercises. Conversely, patients with risk factors for postoperative shoulder stiffness require earlier mobilization to prevent this complication. This group includes patients with coexisting calcific tendinitis, adhesive capsulitis, partial articular supraspinatus tendon avulsion (PASTA) -type rotator cuff repair, concomitant labral repair, and single-tendon rotator cuff repair. Also patients with pre-existing diabetes should start motion early to prevent stiffness. Furthermore, any successful rehabilitation program also needs to be evaluation-based to take into account not only histological healing time lines but also the attainment of specific clinical goals. There is significant variability between the recovery times of patients who have undergone rotator cuff repair. Lastly, for any rehabilitation protocol to succeed, the concept of "Pre-habilitation" needs to be addressed with the patient. This entails having a lengthy discussion with the patient in conjunction their physiotherapist in the preoperative period to cover every aspect of their post-operative recovery and return to function. Educating and preparing the patient regarding their postoperative rehabilitation will only make it easier for them to embrace and comply with your rehabilitation protocol. Pre-habilitation also involves preoperative ROM exercises to maximize shoulder strength of deltoid, intact cuff muscles and scapula stabilizers.

Standard Rehabilitation Program

There are four commonly used and accepted phases of shoulder rehabilitation. The four phases of rehabilitation begin with maintaining and protecting the repair in the immediate postoperative period, followed by progression from early passive range of motion through to return to preoperative levels of function.

Phase I: Passive ROM (Week 1-6)

The goals of this initial phase are to maintain the integrity of the repair without overstress, gradually increase passive ROM, diminish pain and inflammation, and prevent muscular inhibition.

Phase I involves abduction sling immobilization and passive exercises that minimize loads across the repair. This is because immediately following the repair; the strength of your repair construct relies heavily on the suture tendon interface, the number of anchors used, and also the ability to reproduce a tension free repair. Then during the initial healing response, growth factors peak around the second to third week, culminating in the weak fibrin clot being replaced by loosely organized type III collagen callus, neither of which can withstand physiologic loads. We recommend immobilizing the arm in slight abduction (45°) during the phase I and II for a couple of reasons. Firstly, it is known that the hypovascular region of the rotator cuff is about 1.5 cm from its insertion on the greater tuberosity. This position of abduction may enhance regional blood flow by preventing the "wringing out" effect in blood vessels to the tendon. Secondly, abduction of the arm reduces the distance between the origin and the insertion of the muscle tendon unit so that passive tension on the repair site will be decreased. We recommend coming out of the sling 3-4 times during the day to perform the passive exercises, such as after each meal, and during a shower. Furthermore, both passive and active motion of the elbow, wrist, and hand is encourage after surgery.

The benefits of early passive motion have been widely described. It is believed that the gradual introduction of repetitive tensile stress during the maturation process may be beneficial in helping the orientation of biomechanically more robust type I collagen fibers. However, Passive ROM exercises should be performed gently and in a controlled manner within a safe range. Certainly end of range pressure (stretching) should be avoided. An example of passive ROM for forward flexion using closed chain exercise are table slides. While seated at a table, place the hand of the affected shoulder on a sliding surface such as a magazine on a table. Slowly slide the affected hand along the table and bring the head down toward the surface of the table until shoulder is in an elevated position relative to the head. Hold at the end for 15 to 20 seconds and repeat 10 times. Patients repeat this 3 times daily. Similarly, passive external and internal rotation can be performed with the help of PVC canes or wand. It should be performed with the arm positioned at 20 to 45 degrees in the plane of the scapula because rotation with the arm in adduction has been shown to increase tension across the repaired tissues.

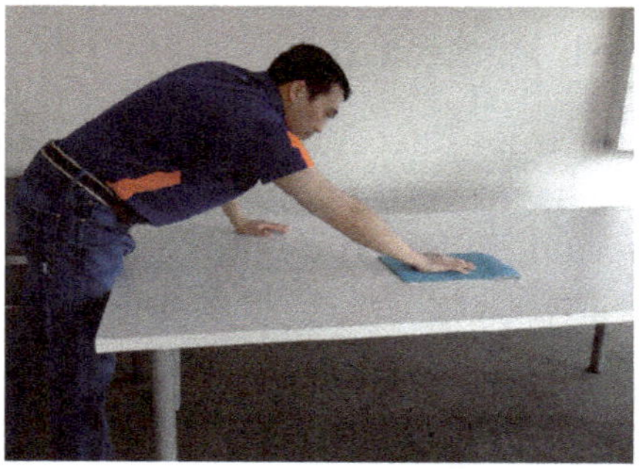

Table slide is performed with the patient leaning over a table and sliding the operative extremity on a piece of paper or a book on a table. Range of motion as tolerated, however it should be limited based on pain.

The use of pulleys is controversial as EMG studies have shown muscle activation and that the rotator cuff is not "quiet" with these activities, so true passive ROM is not achieved. Excessive adduction or internal rotation is avoided because these will place excessive stress on the repair. In the same way, excessive external rotation beyond 20 degrees (maximum excursion in ER should be tested intraoperativey) should be avoided if the subscapularis tear has been repaired. Pendulum exercises can also form part of the passive ROM regimen, as it generates less than 15% of maximum voluntary isometric contraction activity in the rotator cuff muscles. This is performed by simply bending over at the waist, balancing with the good arm on a chair and let the affected arm hang and swing with gravity while drawing concentric circles of about 20 cm diameter. Aquatherapy can be introduced at this time and can be a useful adjunct once the surgical incisions have healed. From weeks 2 to 6, gentle stretching and passive motion can be performed in a pool, 2 to 3 days per week, for 15 to 20 minutes per session. Lastly, it is important to maintain good postural control of scapular and cervical muscles, as well as come out of the sling to perform active ROM of the elbow, wrist and hand to keep them supple.

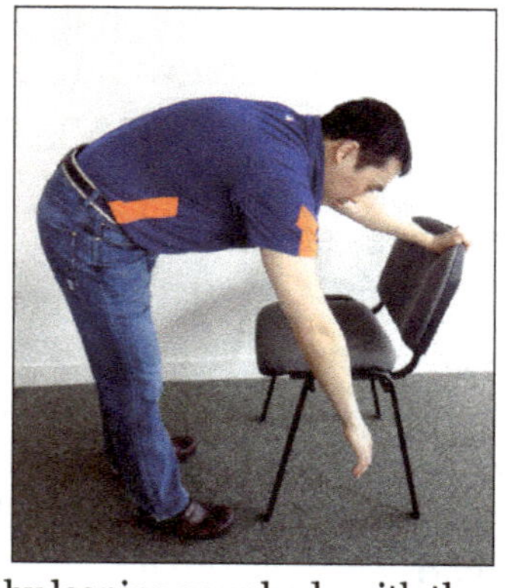

Pendulum exercises performed by leaning your body with the support of a chair and have your arm dangle in front of your body. Both clockwise and counter clockwise motion is performed.

Recommendations:

- Abduction pillow shoulder immobilizer for 6 weeks (4 weeks for partial or small to medium sized <3cm rotator cuff tendon tears with stable surgical fixation).
- Passive supine ROM:
    - Flexion to tolerance 0-140 degrees using table slides.
    - ER and IR in scapular plane 20 to 45 degrees with the use of a wand or cane 4 times a day with 20 repetition.

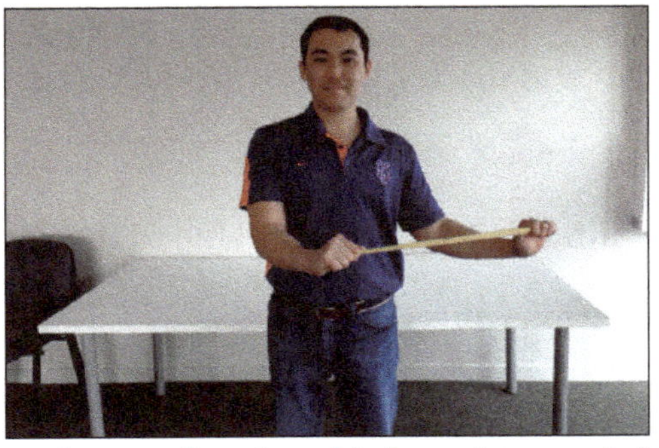

External and internal range of motion with the assistance of a hand wand, stick, or a cane. This exercise should be performed in the plane of the scapula.

Pendulum exercises:

- Active elbow, wrist and hand gripping and ROM.
- Scapular depression and retraction (sitting).
- Neck/upper quarter stretching.
- Cryotherapy for pain and inflammation (ice 15-20 minutes every hour).
- Sleeping (in sling and brace): Usually more comfortable for the patient during the first few weeks postoperative to sleep in a recliner with a pillow underneath the operative extremity while wearing the abduction sling.
- Neuro-muscular re-education (to prevent shoulder/scapular hiking).
- Aquatherapy (week 2-6).
    - 3 times as week for 20 minutes each session.

Precautions:

- No heavy lifting of objects.
- No pushing and pulling.

- No excessive shoulder extension.
- No excessive behind the back movements.
- No excessive stretching or sudden movements.
- No supporting of body weight by hands with transfers in and out of bed and chair.
- No leaning on the elbow.
- Avoid sleeping on the affected side.
- Keep incisions clean and dry for the first week. May shower in 5 to 7 days.

Criteria to progress to next phase:

- Symmetrical and pain free ROM comparable to the contralateral arm.
- If the contralateral arm is affected.
    - Passive forward flexion to at least 125 degrees.
    - Passive external rotation in scapular plane to at least 45 degrees.
    - Passive internal rotation in scapular plane to at least 45 degrees.
    - Passive glenohumeral abduction to at least 90 degrees in the scapular plane.

Phase 2: Active Range of Motion (6 to 12 Weeks)

By 6 weeks postoperatively, most of the acute repair and inflammation processes in the healing phase would have progressed to the collagen remodeling stage. Tendon healing to bone is progressive increasing and able to withstand applied muscle forces generated by simply raising the arm. This low-level active muscle loading help with establishing the orientation of collagen fibres during their maturation stage, which ultimately leading to increased overall tensile strength of the repair construct. Furthermore, active ROM will increase muscle activity and help restore normal patterns of muscle contraction that will enable return to function and allow normal activities of daily living.

The use of pulleys, canes, active assisted ROM (AAROM), and self-assisted ROM however are appropriate at this point. A pillow or towel roll may be used under the arm to help alleviate passive tension across the rotator cuff. This is slowly graduated to full active ROM. It is still advisable to avoid resistance work because tendon-tobone healing strength at this time point is inadequate to withstand the forces generated during strengthening exercises. An example of AAROM includes supine glenohumeral external and internal rotation with stick assistance, as well as supine flexion with the assistance of the uninvolved limb. An alternative AAROM technique is having the patient perform closed chain exercises by drawing circles on a physioball placed on a table with the hand and forearm resting on the ball. In addition, sub-maximal isometric external and internal rotation can be initiated at this time. This involves holding the arm below shoulder height, elbow flexed to approximately 90 degrees, held in a neutral rotation position with a towel roll placed between the elbow and trunk. The patient is asked to generate a force into internal rotation or external rotation, resisting with their uninvolved upper extremity, starting at approximately 25% of maximal effort and gradually increasing to 50-75% of maximal effort without reproducing pain. Open chain proprioceptive exercises help to both restore muscle strength and proprioception, thereby establishing muscular balance. These are performed with the patient lying supine with the involved shoulder held in 90° of forward elevation. The patient is then instructed to draw circles and the alphabet in the air utilizing small, controlled motions.

The scapula-thoracic articulation also should continue to be a focus of therapy as it will allow for the optimal neuromuscular control required for maximal pain free ROM to be achieved. Exercises include shoulder shrugs and scapular retraction. Lying in a prone position can also help initiate proper muscle fiber activity patterns in the rhomboids and trapezius muscles. Then switching to the supine position, the serratus anterior muscle activity can be initiated with scapular protraction in 90 degrees of glenohumeral joint flexion, which is progressed to protraction at 120 degrees of flexion.

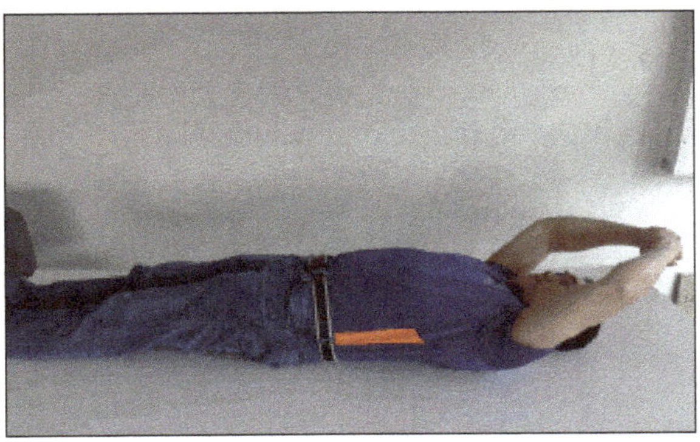

Supine active assisted forward flexion exercise done with the help of the contra-lateral normal arm. Range of motion as tolerated and limited by pain.

Scapular plane elevation (scaption) with a flexed elbow, also known as "the salute exercise", is useful in initiating supraspinatus muscle activity. This exercise can be progressed to "the full can activity", which is known to exhibit high supraspinatus muscle activity.

At 6 to 8 weeks postoperatively, aquatherapy can usually be advanced with the addition of active motion. In our experience, at 10 to 12 weeks the patient can do underwater resistance exercises. Aquatherapy is considered to be active-assisted ROM in a gravity reduced environment. It has been shown that shoulder elevation in the water results in a markedly lower activation of the rotator cuff compared with dry land exercise. This decreased muscle activation during exercise in water should allow for earlier active motion in the postoperative period without compromising the integrity of the repair.

Recommendations:

- Continued passive ROM.
- Introduction of active assisted ROM.
- Patient-directed, self assisted therapy using overhead pulley and stick-assistance methods.
- Open chain proprioceptive exercises.
- Sub-maximal isometric external and internal rotation exercises.
- Ongoing aquatherapy.
- Scapula-thoracic exercises.
- Functional use of the arm for activities of daily living.

Restrictions:

- No resistance or strength activities.

Criteria to progress to next phase:

- Full active ROM compared to the contralateral arm.
- No scapular-thoracic dyskinesia.

Self Directed Home Exercises

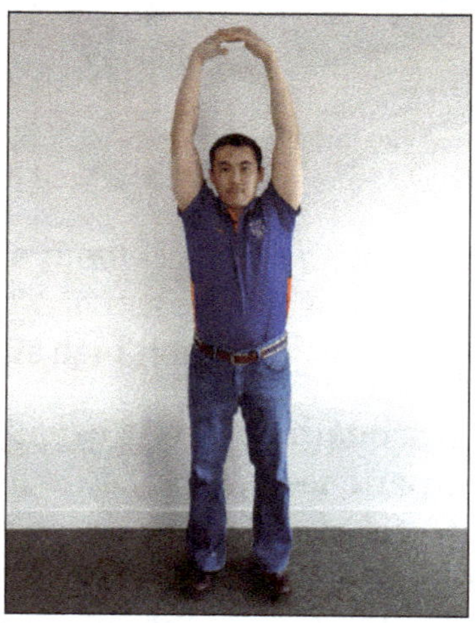

Elbows extending to maximize flexion.

Several active assisted range of motion exercises that the patient can perform at home include using the normal arm to assist and elevate the operative extremity to bring to the top of the head. Then the elbows are extended to increase flexion. This can also be performed with the hand behind the head to increase external rotation. There exercises should be done at home on a regular basis during this phase of therapy.

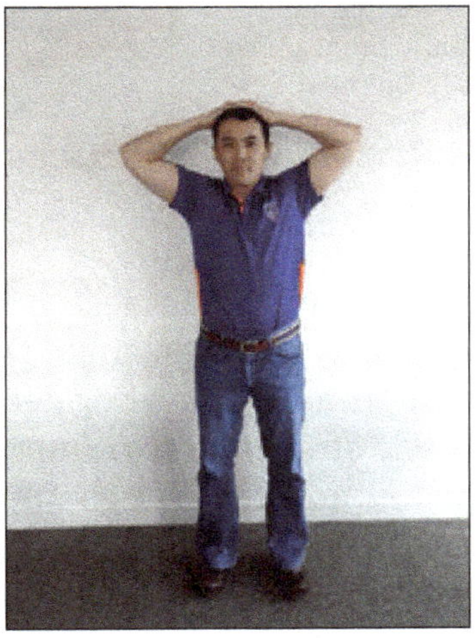

Hand on the top of head with active assistance from the normal contra-lateral arm.

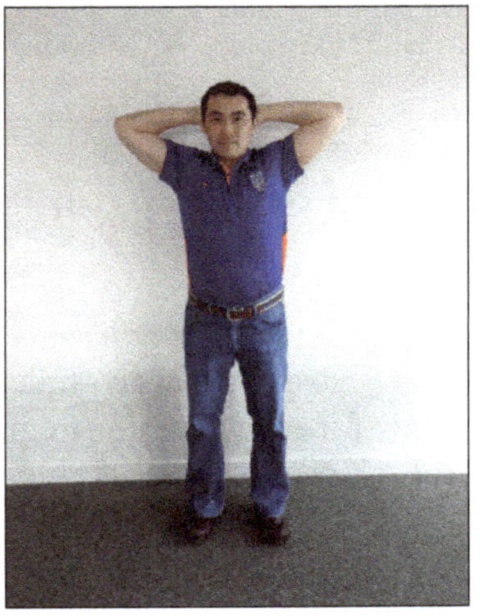

Both hands behind the head to maximize external rotation.

Table: Available clinical evidence in literature for post-operative rehabilitation after rotator cuff repair.

Regimens/method	Outcomes	Complications
All Full thickness RC repair Early group had passive elevation and rotation day 2 Delayed group same protocol at 6 weeks	Both groups similar functional outcomes at 1 year	Slightly higher healing rate in delayed group (91vs85%)
Small to Medium tears Early passive ROM in 1st 4-5 weeks vs No passive	No difference at 12 months for ROM, functional score and VAS	Re-tear 12% of Early passive and 18% of no passive
Medium to Large tears Aggressive group had twice daily manual therapy in 1st 6weeks with unlimited stretching Limited group had limited CPM	Aggressive group had better ROM at 3 months but no difference at 1 year except IR	23.3% retear in aggressive group compared to 8.8% in early limited group
Immediate passive motion or strict immobilization for 6 weeks	Immediate passive motion had better functional scores, less CRPS and less adhesive capsulitis	No difference in healing
N/A	CPM improved ROM in two studies. One study found a decrease in pain and one study found improvement in muscle strength.	N/A

4 week CPM regimen vs manual passive ROM	No difference in functional scores, pain, ROM or isometric strength	N/A
Included all shoulder postop patients including stabilization, arthroplasty and cuff repair	Cryotherapy group had less pain and slept better on the night of surgery. At day 10, less pain and swelling, easier rehab	N/A
Combined aquatic and land-based program vs. land based only	Both improved ROM and functional score. Aquatic program had early better flexion but no difference at 12 weeks	N/A

Phase 3: Initial Strengthening (12 to 16 Weeks)

The strengthening phase should begin approximately 10 to 12 weeks postoperatively depending on the size of the tear, surgical fixation, and patient factors. Histologically, the remodeling phase is nearly complete, with tendon-to bone healing generally strong enough to allow for a graduated program of muscle strengthening. Importantly, both glenohumeral and scapulothoracic kinematics, as well as soft-tissue compliance, should be optimized so that a strengthening program can be safely initiated without pain and in proper form. Attempts to strengthen a stiff shoulder can cause pain, subacromial impingement, and excessive stress on the repair. Only when shoulder mobility or range of motion is maximized are advanced strengthening exercises permitted to increase muscular load. It is important avoid any overhead activity that will result in subacromial contact to occur. Such contact will only exacerbate impingement or stress the repair. Thus, initial exercising of the internal and external rotators should be performed with the arm below the level of the shoulder.

During the initial phase of strengthening, isometric exercises safely allow the controlled application of forces across the tendons without risk of damage. These exercises usually are safe to start early for the periscapular muscles, deltoid, and trapezius because they do not stress the repaired tendons. The second phase of strengthening begins with elastic resistance exercises, concentrating on high repetitions with moderate resistance. The goal of these exercises is to build muscle endurance. The four key exercises are external rotation (infraspinatus, teres minor), internal rotation (subscapularis), forward flexion (anterior deltoid, supraspinatus), and rowing motion (posterior deltoid, periscapular muscles). These exercises are performed with a towel roll placed between the arm and trunk to encourage proper technique, thereby minimizing substitution patterns. More advanced exercises are added as tolerated for the parascapular muscles. To strengthen the serratus anterior muscle, a bear hug exercise using elastic resistance is performed by mimicking a hugging motion around a cylindrical object with the shoulder internally rotated to 45 degrees. To strengthen the trapezius and rhomboid musculature, the standing sport cord row exercise is used. To strengthen the biceps and triceps brachii muscles, conventional biceps curl and triceps extension exercises are used with either isotonic free weight resistance or elastic tubing.

Gradually, advanced proprioceptive and neuromuscular activities are introduced in preparation for light sports activity. These include golf chipping or putting. Any exercise that causes pain, stiffness, or swelling should be discontinued. A core-strengthening program to build up the abdominal musculature is also encouraged.

Recommendations:

- Continue with passive ROM exercises and stretching.
- Continue with self directed home programs and stretching.
- Progressive strengthening (both concentric and eccentric, using safe motions).
- Elastic resistance exercises.
- Parascapular muscle strengthening.
- Core muscle strengthening.
- Advanced proprioceptive and neuromuscular activities in preparation for light sports activity (eg, golf chipping/putting) as tolerated.

Restrictions:

- Avoid overhead activity.

Criteria to progress to next phase:

- Painfree functional ROM with activities of daily living.

Phase 4: Advanced Strengthening (16 to 22 Weeks)

During Phase 4, histologically, the remodeling phase should be complete with the formation of mature collagen robust enough to withstand greater forces. The advanced strengthening phase, is essentially a progression of phase 3 and serves as a transition to sports specific rehabilitation activities. Advanced strengthening of rotator cuff muscles can be strengthened in a number of ways. To isolate infraspinatus and teres minor, perform external rotation exercises of the shoulder at 45 degrees of abduction utilizing elastic resistance while in a standing position. Then, to activate supraspinatus muscle activity, perform external rotation exercises at 90 degrees of abduction. Once again, it is important not to neglect the parascapular muscles as they play an important role in scapulothoracic kinematics. Advanced strengthening of the serratus anterior can be accomplished with exercises such as the pushup with a plus progression from a wall, to a chair, then finally to the floor.

Towards the end of this phase, upper limb plyometrics can be initiated under close supervision. Also known as "jump training" or "plyos", these are exercises based around having muscles exert maximum force in as short a time as possible, with the goal of increasing both speed and power, thereby simulating a sporting environment more closely. It is thought to enhance neuromuscular control, strength and proprioception. An example would include a patient throwing and catching a weighted ball (2 to 10 pounds) against a wall, starting at shoulder height and progressing gradually to overhead.

Recommendations:

- Advanced rotator cuff strengthening, especially of the posterior cuff.
- Continued parascapular muscle training and strengthening.
- Plyometrics.

Restrictions:

- No overhead lifting.
- Not to return to competitive sport until completion of sports rebilitation and internal training.

Criteria to progress to next phase:

- Symmetrical ROM and strength.
- Normalized scapulothoracic kinematics.
- No pain at rest or with activities.

Return to Sports (6 Months)

Prior to a patient being cleared to resume full competitive sports, they must progress through and complete interval sport programs. These are essentially rehabilitation guidelines that simulate sports and recreational activities. They are intended to safely return an athlete to competition as soon as possible while progressively applying appropriate forces to healing structures. Patients who are not athletes still benefit from a functional progression that simulates activities of daily living and work-specific activity. It is recommended that these intensive sports programs should only start after an athlete has completed an adequate cardiovascular warm up prior. The program should be performed three times per week with at least one rest day in-between sessions. To progress to the next level the patient must be able to demonstrate the prior level without pain or limitations. A maintenance exercise program focusing on cardiovascular endurance and flexibility along with scapulothoracic, rotator cuff, lower extremity, and core strength should be performed on alternate days. The same idea can also be applied to criteria for return to work. Depending on the type of work (desk job vs. heavy manual labor), the patient should return when comfortable, pain free, and is able to perform the duties without detriment to the rehabilitation protocol. Manual laborers should only return to work when they have completed all 4 phases of the therapy and have acquired similar range of motion and strength when compared to the normal contra-lateral extremity.

Lumbar Spine Pain

Lumbar spine pain accounts for 5 to 8% of athletic injuries. Although back pain is not the most common injury, it is one of the most challenging for the sports physician to diagnose and treat. Factors predisposing the young athlete to back injury include the growth spurt, abrupt increases in training intensity or frequency, improper technique, unsuitable sports equipment, and leg-length inequality. Poor strength of the back extensor and abdominal musculature, and inflexibility of the lumbar spine, hamstrings and hip flexor muscles may contribute to chronic low back pain. Excessive lifting and twisting may produce sprains and strains, the most common cause of low back pain in adolescents. Blows to the spine may create contusions or fractures. Fractures in adolescents from severe trauma include compression fracture, comminuted fracture, fracture of the growth plate at the vertebral end plate, lumbar transverse process fracture, and a fracture of the spinous process. Athletes who participate in sports involving repeated and forceful hyperextension of the spine may suffer from lumbar facet syndrome, spondylolysis, or spondylolisthesis. The large sacroiliac joint is also prone to irritation. The signs and symptoms of disc herniation in adolescents may be more subtle than in adults. Disorders simulating athletic injury include tumours and inflammatory connective tissue disease. Often, however, a specific diagnosis cannot be made in the young athlete with a low back injury due to the lack of pain localisation and the anatomic complexity of the lumbar spine. A thorough history and physical examination are usually more productive in determining a diagnosis and guiding treatment than imaging techniques. Diagnostic tests may be considered, though, for the adolescent athlete whose back pain is severe, was caused by acute trauma, or fails to improve with conservative therapy after several weeks. Radiographs, bone scanning, computed tomography, and magnetic resonance imaging may help identify, or exclude serious pathology. Fortunately, the majority of cases of low back pain in adolescents respond to conservative therapy. Immediate treatment of an acute injury, such as a sprain or strain, includes cryotherapy, electrogalvanic stimulation, anti-inflammatory medications and gentle exercises. Prolonged bed rest should be avoided since atrophy may occur rapidly. Strong analgesics are also usually contraindicated, except for sleep, since they mask pain and may allow overvigorous activity. Early strengthening exercises include the Williams flexion exercises and/or McKenzie extension exercises. Both exercise motions may often be prescribed. Athletes with an acute disc herniation, however, should only perform extension exercises initially. Athletes with spondylolysis, spondylolisthesis and facet joint irritation should initially be limited to flexion exercises.

When athletes have lower back pain, it can impact their ability to be active and participate in sports, as well as cause pain during every day tasks.

Pain that radiates from the tailbone area down into the thighs often indicates there might be an injury in the athlete's lower back.

Lower Back Pain Risk Factors and Causes in Sports

Almost everyone is at risk of having lower back pain at some point in their life, regardless of whether or not you play sports.

If you play a sport, certain motions may put strain on your back muscles and cause pain.

Other factors that can cause lower back pain include:

- Overuse.
- Being overweight.
- Having poor posture.
- Sitting in a poorly designed chair for a long time.
- A misalignment in the bones of your spine, or vertebrae.
- Arthritis in the spine.
- A small fracture, in rare cases.

Lower Back Pain Complications

Any type of pain can lessen your enjoyment daily activities. If you play a sport, lower back pain can limit your playing time. Athletes can cause strain on other parts of their body if the change the way they walk, lift, swing, or throw to reduce back pain.

Sports that have higher rates of back pain include gymnastics, diving, weight lifting, golf, American football, and rowing. In gymnastics, the incidence of back injuries is 11%. In football linemen, it may be as high as 50%. Ninety percent of all injuries of professional golfers involve the neck or back. Injury rates for 15- and 16-year-old girls in gymnastics, dance, or gym training are higher than the general population, while cross-country skiing and aerobics are associated with a lower prevalence of low back pain. For boys, volleyball, gymnastics, weight lifting, downhill skiing, and snowboarding are associated with higher prevalence of low back pain, while cross-country skiing and aerobics show a lower prevalence.

Back pain is a symptom and has many causes. Muscle strains, ligament sprains, and soft tissue contusions account for as much as 97% of back pain in the general adult population. The majority of athletes with low back pain have a benign source of pain. Muscle strain may be the most common cause of low back pain in college athletes.

The clinical spectrum of spondylolysis, spondylolisthesis, and pars interarticularis stress fractures may be the most common cause of low back pain in adolescents.

Repetitive hyperextension of the low back (gymnastics, figure skating, diving, and football linemen) is a risk factor for the development of spondylolysis.

Hyperlordosis (lordotic low back pain) is the second most common cause of adolescent low back pain. This condition is related to adolescent growth spurts when the axial skeleton grows faster than the surrounding soft tissue, resulting in muscular pain. Other causes of low back pain unique to children are vertebral endplate fractures and bacterial infection of the vertebral disk. Adolescents have weaker cartilage in the endplate of the outer annulus fibrosis, allowing avulsion and resulting in symptoms similar to a herniated vertebral disk. Additionally, the pediatric lumbar spine has blood vessels that traverse the vertebral bodies and supply the vertebral disk, increasing the chance of developing diskitis.

Treatment Options

Cold versus Heat

Cold can be applied to the low back with towels, gel packs, ice packs, and ice massage. Heat methods include water bottles and baths, soft packs, saunas, steam, wraps, and electric pads. There are few high-quality randomized controlled trials supporting superficial cold or heat therapy for the treatment of acute or subacute low back pain. A review cited moderate evidence supporting superficial heat therapy as reducing pain and disability in patients with acute and subacute low back pain, with the addition of exercise further reducing pain and improved function. The effects of superficial heat seem strongest for the first week following injury.

Ultrasound

There are no systemic reviews for ultrasound. One small nonrandomized trial for patients with acute sciatica found ultrasonography superior to sham ultrasonography or analgesics for relief of pain. All patients were prescribed bed rest. For patients with chronic back pain, the small trials were contradictory to whether ultrasonography was any better than sham ultrasonography.

Laser

Low-level laser therapy (LLLT) is a noninvasive light source treatment that generates a single wavelength of light without generating heat, sound, or vibration. Also called *photobiology* or *biostimulation*, LLLT may accelerate connective tissue repair and serve as an anti-inflammatory agent. Wavelengths from 632 to 904 nm are used in the treatment of musculoskeletal disorders. A review of 7 small studies with a total of 384 patients with nonspecific low back pain of varying durations found insufficient data to either support or refute the effectiveness of LLLT for the treatment of low back pain. Because of the varied length of treatment, LLLT dose, application techniques, and different populations, it was not possible to determine optimal administration of LLLT. No side effects were reported.

A recent double-blind randomized placebo-controlled study of 546 patients with acute low back pain (less than 4 weeks) with radiculopathy compared LLLT and nimesulide to nimesulide alone to sham LLLT. Treatment with LLLT and nimesulide improved movement, with more significant reduction in pain intensity and disability and with improvement in quality of life, compared with patients treated only with drugs or placebo LLLT.

Manipulation: Chiropractic, Osteopathic and Manual Physical Therapy

Three systemic reviews analyzed spinal manipulation therapy (SMT) for low back pain, including (1) high-velocity, low-amplitude manipulation of the spinal joints slightly beyond their passive range of motion; (2) high-velocity, low-amplitude technique rotating the thigh and leg; (3) mobilization within passive range of motion; and (4) instrument-based manipulations. There is moderate evidence of short-term pain relief with acute low back pain treated with SMT. Chronic low back pain showed moderate improvement with SMT, which is as effective as NSAIDs and more effective than physical therapy in the long term. Patients with mixed acute and chronic low back pain had better pain outcomes in the short and long terms compared with McKenzie therapy, medical care, management by physical therapists, soft tissue treatment, and back school. SMT was more effective in reducing pain and improving daily activities when compared with sham therapy. Dagenais found SMT effective in pain reduction in the short-, intermediate-, and long-term management of acute low back pain. However, a review in 2004 on SMT in acute and chronic low back pain concluded that there was no difference in pain reduction or ability to perform daily activities with SMT or standard treatments (medications, physical therapy, exercises, back school, or the care of a general practitioner).

Acupuncture

Thirty-five randomized controlled trials did not allow firm conclusions for the effectiveness of acupuncture for acute low back pain. For chronic low back pain, acupuncture is more effective for pain relief and functional improvement than no treatment or sham treatment in the short term only. Acupuncture is not more effective than other conventional or alternative treatments.

Massage

Massage might be beneficial for patients with subacute and chronic nonspecific low back pain, especially when combined with exercises and education. Acupressure or pressure point massage technique was more effective than classic massage. A second systemic review found insufficient evidence to determine efficacy of massage for acute low back pain. Evidence was insufficient to determine effects of the number or duration of massage sessions.

Traction

A meta-analysis found traction no more effective than placebo, sham, or no treatment for any outcome for low back pain with or without sciatica. The results consistently indicated that continuous or intermittent traction as a single treatment for low back pain is not effective. Side effects included worsening of signs and symptoms and increased subsequent surgery; however, the reports are inconsistent.

Transcutaneous Electrical Nerve Stimulation

Evidence from the small number of placebo-controlled trials does not support the use of transcutaneous electrical nerve stimulation in the routine management of chronic low back pain. Evidence from single lower quality trials is insufficient to accurately judge efficacy of transcutaneous electrical nerve stimulation versus other interventions for chronic low back pain or acute low back pain.

Bracing/Lumbar Supports

Braces are not effective in preventing back pain. However, there is conflicting evidence to whether braces are effective supplements to other preventive interventions. Bracing, in combination with activity restriction, is effective in the treatment of spondylolysis in adolescents. A meta-analysis of 15 observational spondylolysis and grade 1 spondylolisthesis treatment studies did not find a significant improvement in rates of healing with bracing when compared with conservative treatment without bracing. Most experts recommend surgical consultation for spondylolisthesis with 50% slippage or more (grade 3 and higher).

Back Schools

There is moderate evidence suggesting that back schools reduce pain and improve function and return-to-work status when compared with exercises, manipulation, myofascial therapy, advice, or placebo. The patients benefiting from back schools had chronic and recurrent nonspecific low back pain in an occupational setting.

Exercise

Exercise therapy appears to be slightly effective at decreasing pain and improving function in adults with chronic low back pain. In subacute low back pain, there is weak evidence that a graded activity program improves absenteeism. In acute low back pain, exercise therapy was no better than no treatment or conservative treatments. Exercise therapy using individualized regimens, supervision, stretching, and strengthening was associated with the best outcomes. The addition of exercise to other noninvasive therapies was associated with small improvements in pain and function.

A randomized single-blind controlled trial compared manual therapy and spinal stabilization rehabilitation to control (education booklet) for chronic back pain. Spinal stabilization rehabilitation was more effective than either manipulation or the education booklet in reducing pain, disability, medication intake, and improving the quality of life for chronic low back pain. A systemic review found segmental stabilizing exercises more effective in reducing the recurrence of pain in acute low back pain; however, exercises were no better than treatment by general practitioner in reducing short-term disability and pain. For chronic low back pain, segmental stabilizing exercises were more effective than treatment from general practitioners but no more effective than exercises using devices, massage, electrotherapy, or heat. In a trial of 30 hockey players, dynamic muscular stabilization techniques (an active approach to stabilization training) were more effective than a combination of ultrasound and short-wave diathermy and lumbar strengthening exercises.

The McKenzie methoduses clinical examination to separate patients with low back pain into subgroups (postural, dysfunction, and derangement) to determine appropriate treatment. The goal is symptom relief through individualized treatment by the patient at home. The McKenzie method is not exclusively extension exercises; it emphasizes patient education to decrease pain quickly, restore function, minimize the number of visits to the clinic, and prevent recurrences. Two systemic reviews have compared the McKenzie method with different conclusions. Clare concluded that McKenzie therapy resulted in decreased short-term (less than 3 months) pain and disability when compared with NSAIDs, educational booklet, back massage with back care advice, strength training with therapist supervision, and spinal mobilization. Machado et alconcluded that the McKenzie method does not produce clinically worthwhile changes in pain and disability when compared with passive therapy and advice to stay active for acute LBP.

A separate review evaluated bed rest versus activity in acute low back pain and sciatica. There were small benefits in pain relief and functional improvement from staying active compared with rest in bed.

Return-to-play

Return-to-play (RTP) guidelines are difficult to standardize for low back pain because of a lack of supporting evidence. A commonly encountered question is, can athletes play through pain? There is no simple answer to this question. For example, an athlete with suspected spondylolysis is generally advised that he or she should not play through pain, while athletes with chronic low back pain from muscular or ligamentous strain may continue to practice, exercise, and compete. However, there is little evidence to support either of these approaches. These athletes should always be monitored for their safety.

Expert opinion guidelines on RTP time frames have been published for lumbar spine conditions. Lumbar strains should achieve full range of motion before RTP. Patients with spondylolysis and spondylolisthesis (grade 1) should rest 4 to 6 weeks and then demonstrate full range of motion and pain-free extension before RTP. Athletes with herniated lumbar disks should rest 6 to 12 weeks following surgical treatment, while those with spinal fusion should wait 1 year to return to activity. Many surgeons advise against return to contact sports following spinal fusion. Iwamoto reviewed conservative and surgical treatments in athletes with lumbar disc herniation and time to return to previous level of sports activity. Seventy-nine percent of conservatively treated athletes returned in an average of 4.7 months, while 85% of those treated with microdiscectomy returned in 5.2 to 5.8 months. Sixty-nine percent of percutaneous discectomies returned in 7 weeks to 12 months.

Sports Concussion

Concussion is an injury risk associated with participation in collision sports. It has been identified as a research priority for many contacts and collision sports governing bodies worldwide. However, concussion remains under-researched in terms of clinical translation from both experimental models to clinical understanding, and from clinical studies to sports policy. Currently, the clinical management of concussion is largely guided by the presence or absence of symptoms with recovery indicated once all post-injury symptoms have resolved. Management of concussion includes physical and cognitive rest until acute symptoms resolve, with a graded program of exertion implemented prior to medical clearance and return-to-play. Considering the potential sequelae, the heterogeneity of symptoms, and the lack of an intervention known to prevent concussion, it is not any wonder that concussion is one of the most complex and perplexing injuries faced by medical professionals, and why making the return-to-play decision can be quite challenging.

Modern sport is a highly competitive and lucrative commercial product, with the health of its major stakeholders, the athletes, regarded as a vital asset. The status of the athlete's cognitive health is an important factor for maintaining a high level of athletic performance and the greatest risk to an athlete's cognitive health in any contact or collision sport, is concussion. In general, sports concussion is recognised as a major health concern worldwide and the management of such injuries is currently one of the most complex topics in sports medicine. Concussion has been increasingly recognised as a large burden of disease and as such has been identified as a research priority for many collision sports' governing bodies worldwide. Despite this concern, concussion is under-researched in terms of clinical translation. Currently, the clinical management of concussion is largely guided by the presence or absence of symptoms with recovery indicated once all post-injury symptoms have resolved. The international guidelines on concussion management and return-to-play recommendations are open to clinician interpretation and based primarily on expert opinion. Until more recently, the management of concussion included physical and cognitive rest until acute symptoms resolve, with a graduated program of exertion implemented prior to medical clearance and return-to-play. Now, complete rest is only considered to be beneficial in the first few days post-concussion, with relative rest and a graduated program of exertion recommended. Considering the heterogeneity of concussion, the differences in presentation between individual athletes, and the lack of an intervention known to prevent concussion, it is clear why concussion is one of the most complex injuries for medical professionals to manage, and how making the return-to-play decision is challenging.

Identification

The identification of a potential concussion is an important initial step in the management process. Removing an athlete from the potential for further harm is thought to reduce an athlete's risk of more serious or catastrophic consequences associated with a second concussion. Importantly, an athlete does not need to be 'diagnosed' with a concussion in order for them to be removed from play, the mantra "if in doubt, sit them out" is quiet frequently quoted and is the conservative approach. In all suspected cases of concussion, the individual should be removed from the playing field and assessed by a physician or licenced healthcare provider. Many sports' governing bodies now have a low threshold for requiring athletes to be removed from play, with 'suspected concussion' providing ample concern that the athlete must be removed from play. Many sporting bodies now apply criteria (identifiable concussion signs) at the elite and semi-professional levels that are considered 'red flags' and require immediate and permanent removal from play, or immediate removal from play and assessment. At all times parents, coaches, and officials need to act in the best interest of athlete safety and welfare by taking responsibility for the recognition, removal, and referral of athletes to a medical doctor.

The Pocket Concussion Recognition Tool was created and updated by the Concussion in Sport Group (CISG; a group of international sports concussion experts) to help identify possible concussion. It is a quick reference and brief tool that may be used to identify suspicion of a concussion through providing a short list of visible cues (of suspected concussion), and signs and symptoms (of suspected concussion), in addition to orientation and memory questions.

Self-reported Symptoms

Athletes may themselves report experiencing a single post-concussion symptom, or a cluster of symptoms that may raise suspicion that a concussion has occurred. These symptoms can be covert (not witnessed by others), whereas other signs may be overt (observed by witnesses). Where an athlete has reported any one of the symptoms presented in table (see for common concussion symptoms), a potential concussion may have occurred and the athlete should be managed conservatively.

Table: Potential symptoms of concussion.

Difficulty remembering	"Do not quite feel right"
Headache	"Pressure in the head"

Confusion	Feeling like "in a fog"
Dizziness	Blurred vision
Sensitivity to light	Sensitivity to noise
Amnesia	Feeling slowed down
Neck pain	Difficulty concentrating
Sadness	More emotional
Nervous or anxious	Fatigue or low energy
Irritability	Nausea

In the Hunter New England Local Health District's Sports Concussion Clinic, the most commonly reported symptoms between 48 and 72 hours post-concussion by the athletes are headache, pressure in the head, dizziness, a general feeling of "not quite being right," and fatigue. Anecdotally, some athletes seem to experience a constellation of symptoms while others do not, which suggests that particular athletes may be more vulnerable to particular post-concussion symptoms than others, and that some symptoms may have an association with others. Many athletes underplay their symptoms in order to return-to-play quicker; this is why objective tests sensitive to post-concussion changes are also an important adjunct to the clinical assessment and certainly to any self-reported symptom questionnaire.

Overt Signs

Overt signs may be witnessed by others such as players, match officials, coaches, managers, other team support staff, parents, and/or fans. Potential symptoms are outlined in table For matches that are televised, the various broadcasters' views are often scrutinised by the expert analysts and the general public at home. The use of video for reviewing a concussion may identify signs of injury that may have been blocked from view or otherwise missed by medical staff. A number of professional contact and collision sports have recently introduced the use of sideline video review for club medical staff to help identify and manage concussions. Numerous studies of video footage have been conducted in a variety of sports; for example, rugby league, rugby union, and Australian rules football. Other sports, such as boxing, soccer, taekwondo, ice hockey, and lacrosse, have also reported on the use of video footage for understanding the circumstances and mechanisms of injury unique to their sports.

Table: Potential signs of concussion.

Loss of consciousness	Blank or vacant stare
Gait ataxia or balance problems	Seizure or convulsion
Clutching or shaking head	Vomiting

Video replay analysis presents a useful tool for sports medicine professionals to identify potential concussions, but it also can be difficult to interpret and presents challenges in identifying those who have sustained a concussion. In a series of work in professional rugby league, the use of video analysis was comprehensively evaluated. Being aware of the combinations of possible concussion signs and the likelihood that various presentations result in a concussion diagnosis can provide a useful addition to sideline concussion identification.

Red Flags

The signs and symptoms of concussion can sometimes be the same as more severe head injuries. It is recommended that more serious action should be taken in the event that there is evidence of loss of consciousness (LOC) or deteriorating conscious state, severe or increasing headache, neck pain, increasing confusion or irritability, repeated vomiting, unusual change in behaviour, or weakness or tingling/burning in the arms or legs. These signs and symptoms are considered to be red flags, and may be an indication of something more serious. If any of these signs/red flags occur, the athlete should immediately attend the nearest Accident and Emergency Centre.

Rugby Union's 'Blue Card' System

World Rugby (the international governing body for the sport of rugby union) introduced a trial 'Blue Card' system across a number of nations over the past few seasons to increase efforts in the identification and management of concussion. The Blue Card initiative provides the on-field referee authority to issue a Blue Card to any player presenting signs of concussion during a match. After receiving a Blue Card, the player must leave the field of play for the remainder of the match and cannot return-to-rugby until they have completed a series of steps designed to ensure they make a full recovery before taking the field again.

Diagnosis

Despite considerable advancement in the field, there still remains an absence of a perfect diagnostic test or marker that can be used by clinicians for an immediate concussion diagnosis. The CISG Berlin Consensus Statement reports that "at present there is no perfect diagnostic test or marker that clinicians can rely on for an immediate diagnosis of concussion". Because a concussion is an evolving process, it is not possible to rule out a concussion when transient neurological symptoms occur. In order to identify and diagnose an injury, a definition is required. There are numerous, varied definitions, but the diagnosis of concussion should always be a medical decision. The Concussion in Sport Group recognises a sports concussion as a traumatic brain injury (TBI) induced by biomechanical forces.

The CISG Berlin, 2016 highlighted that there are a number of features that can be considered in clinically defining concussion:

- Concussion may be caused either by a direct blow to the head, face, neck, or elsewhere on the body with an impulsive force transmitted to the head.

- Concussion typically results in the rapid onset of short-lived impairment of neurological function that resolves spontaneously. However, in some cases, signs and symptoms evolve over a number of minutes to hours.
- Concussion may result in neuropathological changes, but the acute clinical signs and symptoms largely reflect a functional disturbance rather than a structural injury and, as such, no abnormality is seen on standard structural neuroimaging studies.
- Concussion results in a range of clinical signs and symptoms that may or may not involve loss of consciousness. Resolution of the clinical and cognitive features typically follows a sequential course. However, in some cases symptoms may be prolonged.
- The clinical signs and symptoms cannot be explained by drug, alcohol, medication use, other injuries (such as cervical injuries, peripheral vestibular dysfunction, etc.), or other comorbidities (e.g., psychological factors or coexisting medical conditions).

The recent consensus statement on concussion in sport clarified that the final determination regarding sport-related concussion diagnosis and fitness to play is a medical decision based on clinical judgement.

Traditionally, loss of consciousness (LOC) was perceived by many professionals as a necessary sign for the diagnosis of concussion and many of the concussion grading scales reflected the duration of LOC as an important categorisation value. Despite this, there was never a clear association between the duration of LOC and prognosis for a good versus a poor recovery. In traumatic brain injury more generally, the association has had greater support at the severe end of the severity spectrum. For example, duration of coma appeared to have some impact on both early functional outcomes at time of discharge and long-term level of disability (GOS scores at 5–7 years post-TBI). It was also shown to be a strong prognostic factor in predicting both functional and occupational long-term outcome. The majority of studies reported an association between the duration of coma and outcome (i.e., the longer the duration of coma, the worse the outcome). More recently research has reported that LOC occurs in less than 10% of sports concussion at the high school, collegiate, and professional levels.

Assessment, Management and Return–to-activity

A multimodal approach to the clinical assessment of concussed athletes is strongly recommended given concussion is a multi-dimensional injury.

There are many underlying conditions that can mimic post-concussion symptoms, in addition to disorders and conditions that can prolong recovery. Therefore it is essential to the interpretation of the presentation and any assessment measures used in the clinical setting, to collect a comprehensive and thorough history of the athlete. In addition, it is important to ensure that the presenting symptoms are not readily explained by other neurological or medical conditions or disorders, and therefore may potentially be treatable. Individuals without known developmental or health problems, no known history of concussion, also report some non-specific concussion-like symptoms in their daily lives. These symptoms can be related to any number of issues like stress; depression; sleep problems; chronic pain; drug and alcohol abuse; pituitary, thyroid, endocrine, or hormone deficiency; and vascular-related disorders (i.e., diabetes, blood pressure issues, cholesterol problems). Pre-morbid learning disorders, behavioural issues, or mental health problems are all known to be the source of a number of the post-concussion symptoms and clusters of symptoms. For example, athletes with Attention Deficit Hyperactivity Disorder (ADHD) or learning problems have a greater lifetime history of concussion, and individuals with a prior history are at increased risk for a future concussion.

Neuropsychological Assessment

Over two decades ago cognitive tests were first introduced into the sports context to assist with the assessment and management of sports concussion. This paradigm has continued to develop, from the traditional pencil paper-based measures to the computer-based platform. The CISG advocated for the use of empirically based measures for the management of concussion, and they identified neuropsychological testing as a "cornerstone of concussion management". The utility of cognitive testing for the assessment and management of sports concussion was first demonstrated by Barth and colleagues, who recognised the inherent variability in individual performance on neuropsychological measures. This resulted in a within-subjects comparison to assess for cognitive change after a concussion. Comparing athletes' baseline (i.e., pre-injury/ pre-season) and post-injury performance allows for detection of relative deficits, as athletes serve as their own controls. This serial assessment model has been widely accepted by researchers and adopted by many, if not most, high school, collegiate, and professional sports programs as an effective measure of evaluating cognitive impairment. Conventional paper-based neuropsychological testing poses several limitations for sports medicine practitioners (e.g., the extensive time requirements for administration, scoring, and interpretation; practice effects from serial presentation of a finite number of stimuli; and floor and ceiling effects). Additionally, the traditional tests were never designed nor validated for serial assessment over brief periods of time. Intent on overcoming such important clinical limitations, computerised adaptations of conventional neuropsychological tests were developed. Computer-based test batteries have been recognised as an effective concussion-screening tool because of their ability to be administered simultaneously to a large group, increased timing accuracy, and decreased practice effects. At this point of time there are a number of commercial computerised neuropsychological tests that are available for athletes at all levels of competition. Two of the most commonly used are ImPACT.

Neuroimaging

Computer tomography (CT) and structural magnetic resonance imaging (MRI) are typically unhelpful in athletes suffering sports concussion beyond ruling out a more severe traumatic brain injury—in individuals where it is potentially clinically indicated. However, advanced neuroimaging techniques have increasingly been used in a research context, with speculation that some of these techniques may translate to the clinical setting. Some research in acutely concussed athletes with advanced neuroimaging techniques have demonstrated an association with metabolic and physiological changes in the brain, which correlate with post-concussive symptoms and performance on cognitive testing.

All of the 76 eligible studies using neuroimaging and/or electrophysiological measures reported significant effects of concussion. This likely reflects the publication bias in the literature (i.e., positive findings are more often published than negative findings), the numerous output variables of these modalities that are available to the researcher for conducting multiple comparisons (which increases the likelihood of false positive findings), or that these modalities are more sensitive to post-concussion changes. There are many issues in attempting to bring the literature together when considering each of these modalities; for example, there are a limited number of studies for any specific marker, varying post-concussion time frames when the data was collected, an absence of any standardised acquisition protocol, or post-processing and analyses.

The majority of task-functional MRI (fMRI) studies use a working memory paradigm, and has resulted in varied findings. Increased and decreased activity in task-related networks (e.g., dorsolateral prefrontal cortex) have been reported. The variability in methodology (i.e., the type and number of stimuli used [low versus high working memory 'load']) may explain apparent discordance in hypoactivation versus hyperactivation results reported. In concussed athletes, activity outside of the core task regions have also been reported in a variety of tasks. Varying methodology is also a considerable limitation in interpreting the resting-state fMRI (rs-fMRI) literature. The default mode network (DMN) is the most extensively studied network in the concussion and rs-fMRI literature, and results have reported both increases and decreases in connectivity between DMN regions. Altered functional connectivity has also been observed relative to executive function, visual, and motor networks. Reduced cerebral blood flow (CBF) has been reported during the acute and sub-acute phases (days to weeks) post-concussion, as well as at more chronic time points (approximately 5 months).

The use of diffusion tensor imaging (DTI) has increased substantially over the past few years. In 2012, a systematic review of the DTI and concussion literature reported on eight studies and raised concern in the literature at the time that there was so much variability in the methodology bringing together the findings of the diverse range of work and attempting to interpret the results was challenging. A more recent DTI and concussion systematic review suggested that the most consistent findings were decreased mean diffusivity and an increase in fractional anisotropy in white matter within

6 months post-concussion, but these findings are not universal (i.e., the opposite patterns have also been reported in other studies). In addition, reduced radial diffusivity has been reported, but increase and decrease in axial diffusivity have been described.

The magnetic resonance spectroscopy (MRS) and sports concussion literature was systematically reviewed in 2013. The review included 11 eligible studies. The reseachers of the systematic review raised concerns regarding the absence of studies examining sensitivity and specificity of MRS for concussion and the lack of longitudinal studies involving a reasonably large cohort of injured athletes. One of the greatest shortcomings, was that there was no way of determining how to interpret reliable or clinically significant changes in neurometabolites in individual athletes, because there were no studies involving test-retest reliability. Unfortunately almost 5 years later, this shortcoming has not been resolved. In addition, there is no consensus pertaining to the ideal methodology, with a variety of methods used to measure metabolite concentrations. The availability of additional metabolites, such as Glutamate (Glu) and myo-inositol (mI), might add to the sensitivity and specificity of MRS measures (as shown in severe traumatic brain injury). Therefore, adoption of short echo time methods or other means of obtaining additional biochemical measures would be advantageous. In general, MRS results have found reduced N-acetylaspartate (NAA; relative to creatine and/or choline) predominately in white matter, with some evidence of acute reduction with subsequent recovery by 30 days post-injury in the MRS literature. There is also evidence that NAA may be decreased more chronically.

Several studies have demonstrated the effects of concussion on electroencephalogram (EEG)/quantitative-EEG (qEEG) at rest or during various task conditions. Measures from qEEG have also been shown to be altered at 8 days post-concussion relative to baseline, and have been associated with concussion severity, underlining the potential of electrophysiological measurements in the assessment of concussion.

In view of the limitations of the literature (e.g., lack of generalisability due to the inclusion of limited age ranges, male athletes focus and limited sample sizes, lack of appropriate control groups, lack of pre-injury enrolment and potential for measurement bias due to limited information regarding the definition/diagnosis of mTBI/SRC), the reseachers of the systematic review on advanced neuroimaging from the CISG Berlin, 2016 suggested that "the level of evidence for the role of these neuroimaging and electrophysiological measures in the clinical assessment of concussion is low because the most studies reviewed were not designed to specifically assess clinical potential." However, the reseachers also suggested that "there is a significant role for neuroimaging and electrophysiological measures in characterising the pathophysiology of concussion".

Blood and Fluid Biomarkers

Blood (plasma or serum), saliva, and cerebral spinal fluid (CSF) have become an increasingly utilised method for analysing various biomarkers post-concussion. Proteomics (the study of proteins) has advanced in such a manner that many researchers and clinicians are becoming increasingly interested in collecting samples from athletes. A recent systematic review reported 11 studies found significant alterations in one or more of the following blood biomarkers that could potentially aid in the diagnosis of concussion: α-amino-3-hydroxy-5-methyl-4-isoxazolepropionic acid receptor peptide (AMPAR), S100 calcium binding protein B (s100B), total tau, marinobufagenin, plasma soluble cellular prion protein, glial fibrillary acidic protein, neuron-specific enolase (NSE), calpain-derived αII-spectrin N-terminal fragment (SNTF), tau-C79, and metabolomics profiling.

Oculomotor and Vestibular Function

The vestibular and oculomotor systems are important in sensing angular and linear acceleration of the head and eyes, which enables a moving individual to maintain gaze on a stable target or a stationary individual to focus on a moving target. Sports concussion clinical researchers have observed vestibular and oculomotor pathway involvement in the recovery from concussion in certain athletes. As such, many concussion-screening programs now include vestibular and oculomotor testing. Vestibular and oculomotor screening may include an assessment of pursuits, saccades, vestibular ocular reflex, visual motion sensitivity, and convergence via symptom provocation and measurement of near-point convergence. Vestibular and oculomotor impairment and symptoms may be associated with worse outcomes after sports concussion, including prolonged recovery. Identifying clinical profiles may help to inform better treatment and earlier intervention to reduce recovery time after concussion. As such, screening for and subsequent monitoring of vestibular and oculomotor impairment and symptoms are critical to assessing and informing subsequent referral, treatment, and return-to-play. Combining these assessments with others that examine whole-body behavioural output of vestibular, visual, and somatosensory integration (e.g., postural balance) may increase sensitivity and greatly improve concussion management. McDevitt and colleagues reported that using a condensed set of balance, and vestibular and oculomotor tests resulted in the greatest accuracy for detecting concussion.

Dual-tasks

Not only has a multimodal approach to the assessment of athletes suffering concussion been endorsed, but the assessment of multiple domains simultaneously has been considered to be more sensitive to post-concussion sequelae as a means of stressing the system. fMRI studies using dual-task paradigms have demonstrated recruitment of many neuroanatomical areas outside of the typical structures known to service certain cognitive functions. In addition, the introduction of a cognitive task while walking has been shown to distinguish concussed from non-concussed athletes and may be used as a paradigm for monitoring recovery post-concussion.

Rest

Many of the original guidelines and consensus and agreement statements for managing sports concussion have recommended that athletes rest until they have made a complete recovery (i.e., symptom free). As such, rest has been almost universally recommended as part of the 'treatment' process. However, 'rest' is a misnomer; it is not possible for an athlete to be at complete rest (both physically and cognitively), so it is more accurate to label the recommendation as 'relative rest.' Rest has been assumed to ease discomfort during the acute recovery period by mitigating post-concussion symptoms and/or that rest may promote recovery by minimising brain energy demands following concussion. The most recent systematic review on rest and treatment conducted by a number of leading clinicians and researchers from the Concussion in Sport Group and the consensus statement reported that "there is currently insufficient evidence that prescribing complete rest achieves these objectives. After a brief period of rest during the acute phase (24–48 hours) after injury, patients can be encouraged to become gradually and progressively more active while staying below their cognitive and physical symptom-exacerbation thresholds (i.e., activity level should not bring on or worsen their symptoms)." Refraining from engaging in vigorous exertion while an athlete is recovering is recommended, however, the extent of exercise and duration of rest, or relative rest, is not yet well defined and requires further study.

The Graduated Return–to-play (GRTP)

The graduated return-to-play (GRTP) is a six-stage program of increased intensity that is completed over a minimum of 6 days (i.e., each stage should take at least 24 hours). If an athlete who is engaged in the GRTP process experiences a return of any post-concussion symptoms, then the athlete is to return to the previous step. In the 2016 consensus statement, the CISG added clarification regarding athletes who experience persisting symptoms (i.e., symptoms lasting more than 10–14 days in adults or more than 1 month in children), stating that the athlete should be referred to a healthcare professional who is an expert in the management of concussion. The CISG also clarified that resistance training should be added only in the later stages (stage 3 or 4 at the earliest). A summary of the GRTP recommendations for each of these stages is presented in table.

Table: Graded return-to-play (GRTP).

Stage	Aim	Activity	Goal of each step
1	Symptom-limited activity	Daily activities that do not provoke symptoms.	Gradual reintroduction of work/ school activities.
2	Light aerobic exercise	Walking or stationary cycling at slow to medium pace. No resistance training.	Increased heart rate.
3	Sport-specific exercise	Running or skating drills. No head impact activities.	Add movement.

4	Non-contact training drills	Harder training drills, for example, passing drills. May start progressive resistance training.	Exercise, coordination and increased thinking.
5	Full contact training	Following medical clearance, participate in normal training activities.	Restore confidence and assess functional skills by coaching staff.
6	Return-to-sport	Normal game play.	

This table has been modified from the CISG Consensus Statement. An initial period of 24–48 hours of both relative physical rest and cognitive rest is recommended before commencing the GRTP process.

Potential Longer Term Concerns

Understanding the possible long-term effects of concussions sustained during a career in contact sports has become an area of considerable interest. Repetitive neurotrauma sustained during a career in boxing has been reported to be associated with chronic brain damage in some former athletes since the 1920s, but it has only been associated with former National Football League (NFL) players more recently. A review on this issue conducted by Manley and colleagues reported that there is emerging evidence that some retired NFL players have mild cognitive impairment, neuroimaging abnormalities, and differences in brain metabolism disproportionate to their age. Autopsy cases of former professional football players (among others also in the sample) have revealed diverse forms of neuropathology, including immunoreactivity for hyperphosphorylated tau (p-tau) in a specific pattern (e.g., irregularly distributed in depths of cortical sulci) in which p-tau is not expected to be present through normal ageing or in association with frontotemporal dementia or Alzheimer's disease.

In view of the speculation pertaining to the possible consequences concussion may have on the health of some athletes later in their life, current athletes often raise concerns regarding the issue of retirement. In the clinical setting, athletes are regularly presenting following a single, or in some instances multiple, Concerned that they are at high-risk of long-term issues. It is not possible at the current time to predict or diagnose CTE in-life. The diagnosis is made through neuropathological examination on autopsy. There are a number of research groups around the world currently conducting prospective, longitudinal studies to further understand this disease, but it will take a generation of players (or longer) to fully comprehend the extent of the issue, and the factors that place some athletes at risk versus others who appear to be resilient. Providing athletes with information to empower them to make a well-informed decision regarding retirement is a complex issue. Currently no evidenced-based, scientifically validated guidelines for forming the basis of such a decision exist. In the absence of strong empirical evidence to support recommendations, clinical decision-making must be individualised and should involve a multidisciplinary team of experts in concussion and traumatic brain injury. Involving a multidisciplinary team enables a thorough investigation of all domains, and where clinical indications are present, it enables all possible differential diagnoses to be appropriately considered.

Ankle Sprains

An ankle sprain is a common injury. Inversion-type, lateral ligament injuries represent approximately 85% of all ankle sprains. The incidence of ankle sprain is highest in sports populations. Poor rehabilitation after an initial sprain increases the chances of this injury recurrence.

The ankle joint is the body part that is second-most likely to be injured in sport. In the United States of America the total cost of ankle sprains is approximately $2billion. A meta-analysis by Doherty et al, found that indoor sports carry the greatest risk of ankle sprain with an incidence of 7 per 1,000 cumulative exposures. Severe ankle sprains occur commonly in basketball players. From a study of elite Australian basketball players, McKay et al, reported that the rate of ankle injury was 3.85 per 1000 participations. Recurrence rates amongst basketball players is reported to be greater than 70%. Athletes with chronic ankle instability miss practices and competition, require ongoing care in order to remain physically active, and display sub-optimal performance.

Of the lateral ankle ligament complex the most frequently damaged one is the anterior talofibular ligament (ATFL). Their anatomical location and the mechanism of sprain injury mean that the calcaneo-fibular (CFL) and posterior talofibular ligaments (PTFL) are less likely to sustain damaging loads.

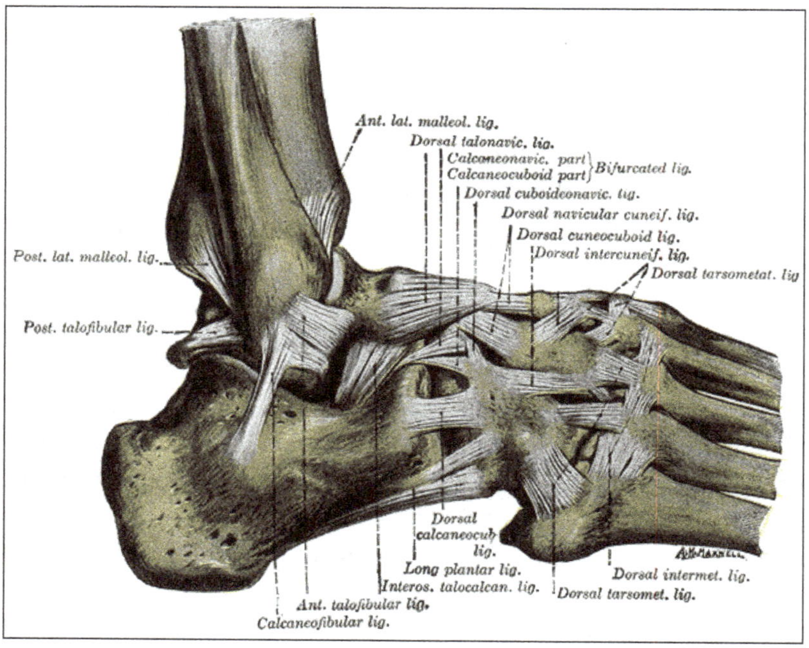

On the medial side the strong, deltoid ligament complex posterior tibiotalar (PTTL), tibiocalcaneal (TCL), tibionavicular (TNL) and anterior tibiotalar ligaments (ATTL)] is injured with forceful "pronation and rotation movements of the hindfoot".

The stabilising ligaments of the distal tibio-fibular syndesmosis are the anterior-inferior, posterior-inferior, and transverse tibio-fibular ligaments, the interosseous membrane and ligament, and the inferior transverse ligament. A syndesmotic (high ankle) sprain occurs with combined external rotation of the leg and dorsiflexion of the ankle.

Risk Factors

Several intrinsic and extrinsic risk factors predispose an athlete to chronic ankle instability. The most common risk factor is previous history of sprain. A previous sprain may compromise the strength and integrity of the stabilisers and interrupt sensory nerve fibres. Sex, height, weight, limb dominance, postural sway and foot anatomy are intrinsic. Extrinsic risk factors may include taping, bracing, shoe type, competition duration and intensity of activity.

Mechanism of Injury/Pathological Process

Lateral ankle sprains usually occur during a rapid shift of body center of mass over the landing or weight-bearing foot. The ankle rolls outward, whilst the foot turns inward causing the lateral ligament to stretch and tear. When a ligament tears or is overstretched its previous elasticity and resilience rarely returns. Some researchers have described situations where return to play is allowed too early, compromising sufficient ligamentous repair Reports have proposed that the greater the level of plantar flexion the higher the likelihood of sprain Yeung et al, 1994, in an epidemiological study of unilateral ankle sprains, reported that the dominant leg is 2.4 times more vulnerable to sprain than the non-dominant one. A less common mechanism of injury involves forceful eversion movement at the ankle injuring the strong deltoid ligament.

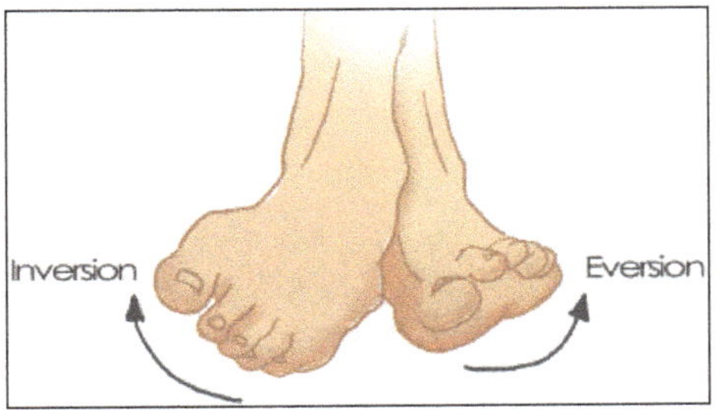

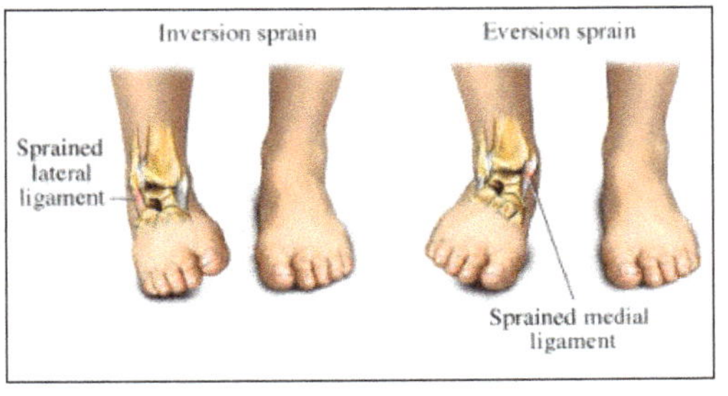

Aspect	Mechanism of injury	Ligaments
Lateral	Inversion and plantarflexion	Anterior talofibular ligament Calcaneo-fibular ligament Posterior talofibular ligament
Medial	Eversion	Posterior tibiotalar ligament Tibiocalcaneal ligament Tibionavicular ligament Anterior tibiotalar ligament

High	External rotation and dorsiflextion	Anterior-inferior tibiofibular ligament Posterior-inferior tibiofibular ligament Transverse tibiofibular ligament Interosseous membrane Interosseous ligament Inferior transverse ligament

Clinical Presentation

- Patient presents with inversion injury or forceful eversion injury to the ankle. May have previous history of ankle injuries or instability.
- Able to partial weight-bear only on the affected side.
- If patient presents with description of cold foot or paraesthesia, suspect neuro-vascular compromise of peroneal nerve.
- Tenderness, swelling and bruising can occur on either side of the ankle.
- No bony tenderness, deformity or crepitus present.
- Passive inversion or plantar flexion with inversion should replicate symptoms for a lateral ligament sprain. Passive eversion should replicate symptoms for a medial ligament sprain.
- Special Tests: +ve Anterior Draw, Talar Tilt or Squeeze Test (depending on the structures involved).

Differential Diagnosis

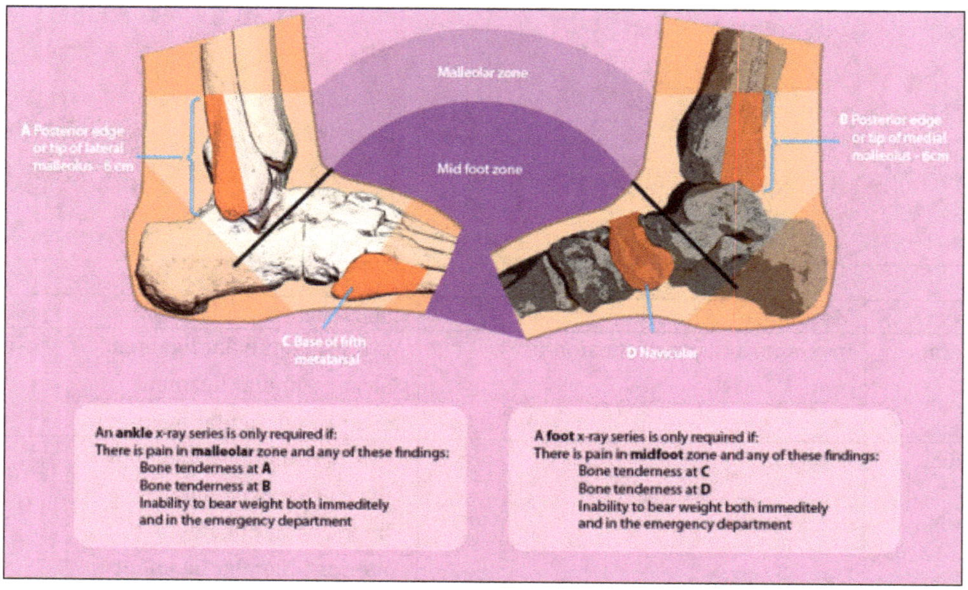

Additional differential diagnosis to look out for:

- Impingement.
- Tarsal Tunnel Syndrome.
- Sinus Tarsi Syndrome.
- Cartilage or psteochondral injuries.
- Peroneal Tendinopathy or subluxation.
- Posterior Tibial Tendon Dysfunction.

Classification Grading Systems

There are numerous grading systems used for the classification of ligament sprains, each having their strengths and weaknesses. Different therapists may employ different systems so effective continuity of care, the patient should see the same therapist each time.

The traditional grading system for ligament injuries focuses on a single ligament

- Grade I represents a microscopic injury without stretching of the ligament on a macroscopic level.
- Grade II has macroscopic stretching, but the ligament remains intact.
- Grade III is a complete rupture of the ligament.

As there are ankle multiple ligaments across the joint it may not be always straight forward to use a grading system that is designed for describing the state of a single ligament unless it is certain that only a single ligament is injured. Some authors have therefore resorted to grading lateral ankle ligament sprains by the number of ligaments injured. It is, however, hard to be certain on the number of ligaments torn unless there is clear, high quality radiographic or surgical evidence.

A third system which can be adopted is a 3 graded classification based on the severity of sprain injury.

- Grade I Mild: Little swelling and tenderness with little impact on function.
- Grade II Moderate: Moderate swelling, pain and impact on function. Reduced proprioception, ROM and instability.
- Grade III Severe: Complete rupture, large swelling, high tenderness loss of function and marked instability.

This scale is largely subjective due to individual therapist interpretation. However, the same can be said for the other classifications unless clear radiographic evidence is available or assessed and treated by surgical intervention.

Rehabilitation of Lateral Ankle Sprains

Lateral ankle sprains are one of the most common injuries in athletes. The rate of injury is as high as 70%. The most commonly involved ligament is the anterior talofibular ligament (ATFL), followed by the calcaneofibular (CFL) and posterior talofibular ligament (PTFL). The common mechanism of injury is inversion with excessive ankle supination in forced plantarflexion when the ankle joint is in its most unstable position. There are three grades of ankle sprains: Grade I, mild with an incomplete tear of ATFL; Grade II, moderate with a complete tear of ATFL with or without an incomplete tear of CFL; and Grade III, severe with complete tear of ATFL and CFL. Grades I and II respond well to functional treatment. Functional treatment includes RICE protocol, i.e., rest, ice, compression, and elevation. It also includes range of motion and strengthening exercises, proprioceptive training, and sports-specific exercises. Bracing and taping of the ankle joint help in preventing the sprains and also reduce the recurrence of the injury. Grade III ankle injury may be treated with surgery if the symptoms persist post functional treatment.

The ankle joint is the most commonly affected joint in sports of which lateral ankle sprains are the most common. The sports in which lateral ankle sprains are a frequent occurrence are football, basketball, running, volleyball, tennis, badminton, ballet/dance, etc. In many sports the rate of injury is as high as 70%. Unilateral ankle sprains are reported in 52%, whereas for bilateral ankle sprains, the number is 48%. The recurrence rate of ankle injury in athletes is 73%. The incidence is high between 15 and 19 years of age with no significant difference in the gender.

Biomechanics

The lateral ankle compartment comprises the anterior talofibular ligament (ATFL), the calcaneofibular ligament (CFL), and the posterior talofibular ligament (PTFL). The most commonly injured ligament is the ATFL as it is the weakest of all three ligaments. In frequency of injury, the ATFL is followed by the calcaneofibular ligament CFL. The PTFL is rarely injured as it is the strongest of all the three ligaments. The most common mechanism of injury in lateral ankle sprains is when, in forced plantar flexion, inversion occurs with excessive ankle supination. In that position the ankle joint is the most unstable. In the course of the inversion, the body's center of gravity moves over the ankle leading to ankle sprains. There are three clinical grades of lateral ankle sprains.

- Grade I—Mild: There is an incomplete tear of ATFL with little swelling and tenderness, minimal or no functional loss, and no mechanical joint instability.
- Grade II—Moderate: Complete tear of ATFL with or without an incomplete tear of CFL with moderate pain, swelling, and tenderness over the involved structures; some joint motion is lost, and joint instability is mild to moderate.

- Grade III—Severe: Complete tears of ATFL and CFL with marked swelling, hemorrhage, and tenderness. There is loss of function, and joint motion and instability are markedly abnormal.

Chronic Ankle Instability (CAI)

Athletes with chronic ankle instability give a history of two or three severe ankle sprains with the main complaint being intermittent giving out of the ankle. The athlete often complains of difficulty and apprehension on uneven surfaces. Even mild exacerbations lead to short-term dysfunction. It is characterized by residual ankle instability as a result of either mechanical ankle stability or functional ankle instability or a combination of both.

Mechanical and Functional Instability

Mechanical instability (MI) and functional instability (FI) are both due to recurrent lateral ankle sprains. Mechanical instability is defined as an increase in the accessory movements in the joint leading to hypermobility. Residual MI usually results from a tear or lengthening of one of the ligamentous structures supporting the joint and suggests a suboptimal healing process after injury. A lesser known phenomenon is hypomobility leading to ankle instability. Joint hypomobility can be intra-articular or extra-articular, giving rise to restricted range of motion at the ankle. Hypomobility occurs at the subtalar, talocrural joint, distal tibiofibular joint, and proximal tibiofibular joint.

As the joint develops MI, proprioceptive changes occur, which result in alterations in defense mechanism to prevent injuries, thus leading to CAI. FI can result in balance deficits, joint position sense deficits, delayed peroneal muscle reaction time, altered common peroneal nerve function, strength deficits, a decreased range of motion (ROM), sinus tarsi syndrome, and anterolateral impingement syndrome.

Rehabilitation

Early mobilization of ankle sprains as compared with cast immobilization has been shown to be more comfortable as it results in less pain and provides for an earlier return to work. Cast immobilization does not improve healing compared with an active mobilization rehabilitation program and may have negative implications in relation to muscle wasting and stiffness. Functional treatment is considered better in achieving more effective mobilization and an earlier return to daily activities. Lateral ankle sprains respond well to the conservative treatment which includes initially RICE—rest, ice, compression, and elevation—followed by early mobilization. Rehabilitation focuses on restoring ROM, strength, balance, and normal gait patterns. Functional rehabilitation begins on the day of injury and continues until pain-free gait and activities are attained. Functional rehabilitation has four aspects: ROM, strengthening, proprioception, and activity-specific training. Ankle joint stability is a prerequisite to the institution of functional rehabilitation. Since Grade I and Grade II injuries are considered stable, functional rehabilitation should begin immediately.

Reduce Pain and Swelling

Rest

Rest is prescribed to avoid undue stress on the joint. It is required to reduce the metabolic demands on the injured tissue and thus avoid increased blood flow. It also helps in avoiding stress on the injured tissue that might disrupt the fragile fibrin bond, which is the first element of the repair process. Rest can be applied selectively to allow some general activity, but athletes must avoid stressful activities.

Ice

Cryotherapy involves a nice bath with a temperature of 4°–10°C for 12–20 min, one to three times per day, and applying an ice pack to the injured area for 15–20 min, one to three times per day. Ice therapy should be started immediately after the injury and ice application initiated within day 0 or day 1. Both have shown better results and return to full activity as compared to when the ice was applied after 48 h. Ice application should provide deep penetration to gain full benefits. Also the ice should not be held immobile in one area or frostbites may occur.

Ice application causes vasoconstriction which decreases blood flow and therefore swelling to the injured area. The lowering of tissue temperature decreases the metabolism and the chemical actions of cells and thus lowers the oxygen and nutrient needs in the affected area. Decreased blood flow limits edema; there is less histamine release and therefore less capillary breakdown than would normally be present after injury. There is better lymphatic drainage from the injured area because of the lower pressure on the extravascular fluid table.

Table: Cryotherapy generates four stages of sensation.

Stage	Duration (min)	Sensation
Stage 1	1–3	A cold feeling is noted.
Stage 2	2–7	Burning or aching.
Stage 3	5–12	Local numbness and anesthesia (decreased conductivity of regional nerve fibers).
Stage 4	12–15	Reflex deep tissue vasodilation without an increase in metabolism.

Hence, the rationale of minimum 15 min of cryotherapy per treatment.

Compression and Elevation

Compression and elevation work better in combination with cryotherapy. Compression with an adhesive bandage and a foot elevation of more than 45° is the standard prescribed treatment for lateral ankle sprains. Compression can also be achieved by both adhesive and nonadhesive tapes, but it is important to renew them timely as the compression wears off with time. Normally a nonadhesive tape should be renewed after

3 days, and an adhesive tape should be renewed after 5 days. This prevents swelling and immobilizes the injured area which prevents further injury and thus promotes healing. Passive exercises can be started in stage 3 which is the local numbness stage in which the athlete experiences less discomfort when exercising.

Improve Range of Motion (ROM)

Range of Motion Exercises

Range of motion exercises include both active and passive exercises. Achilles tendon stretching should be started within 48–72 h in a pain-free range irrespective of weight-bearing status of the athlete to avoid the tissue from contracting. Self-passive stretches can also be given with the help of a towel. Next, the stretches should be extended to weight-bearing position, which can be done by standing on an inclined surface and asking the athlete to shift his/her weight forward. The stretches should be maintained 15–30 s, repeated 10 times, and should be done 3–5 times per day. Passive exercises are followed by active ROM exercises whereby the athlete can do alphabet letter exercises, i.e., drawing letters in the air both in upper and lower cases. The exercises should be done 2–3 times per hour, 4–5 times per day. Stationary biking can also be included to improve dorsiflexion and plantar flexion motion in a controlled environment while providing a cardiovascular workout for the athlete.

Manual Therapy

Manual therapy is started within 48 h after the injury when ankle dorsiflexion is restricted. To improve range, a gentle oscillating passive joint mobilization is given. Here the talus is moved posteriorly. By the convex concave rule, when the talus is moved posteriorly, the convex talus rolls upward and slides posteriorly on the concave surface of the crux, thus improving the dorsiflexion range. In a technique described by Maitland, with the athlete in supine position, the affected foot is taken in the available pain-free ROM in dorsiflexion. Gentle oscillations are then given to the joint to avoid pain and spasm. The oscillations are given for 60 s, 2 or more times with a rest of 10 s taken in between.

Mobilization with movement is another technique of manual therapy suggested by Mulligan which helps with increasing the ROM actively. In this technique the athlete position is high kneeling with weight-bearing on the affected limb or standing with the affected foot placed forward. In both positions the ankle is in neutral position. A padded belt is used for mobilization and is placed in such a way that the bottom of the belt is leveled with the inferior margin of the medial malleolus. The position of the mobilization belt allows the examiner to fix the talus and calcaneus with his/her hands and draws the tibia forward on the talus, thereby creating a relative posterior talar glide. Once the glide is given, the athlete actively dorsiflexes the ankle in a pain-free range. The glide should be maintained throughout the movement. Two sets of 10 repetitions, separated by a 2-min rest, are performed. Once ROM is achieved and swelling and pain are controlled, the athlete is ready to proceed to the strengthening phase of rehabilitation.

Improve Strength

Strengthening of weakened muscles is essential for a quick recovery and thus helps in preventing re-injury. An eversion to inversion strength ratio >1.0 is an important indicator of ankle sprain injury. Exercises should focus on strengthening the peroneal muscles because insufficient strength in this group of muscles has been associated with CAI and recurrent injury. However, all muscles of the ankle should be targeted, and all exercises should be performed bilaterally. When the training is performed bilaterally, we can expect substantial strength gains in both extremities. Strengthening begins with isometric exercises performed against an immovable object in four directions of ankle movement and is progressed to dynamic resistive exercises (isotonic exercises) using ankle weights, surgical tubing, or resistance bands.

With a structured rehabilitation program, the athlete can create continuous goals and more easily appreciate improvements. A daily adjustable progressive resistance exercise (DAPRE) strength progression, originally described by Knight and later modified by Perrin and Gieck, can be used to create a structured progression of exercises for the athletes. The strengthening exercises should be performed with an emphasis on the eccentric component. Athletes should be instructed to pause 1 s between the concentric and eccentric phases of exercise and perform the eccentric component over a 4-s period. Concentric contraction refers to the active shortening of the muscle with resultant lengthening of the resistance band, while eccentric contraction involves the passive lengthening of the muscle by the elastic pull of the band. Resistive exercises should be performed (2–3 sets of 10–12 repetitions) in all four directions twice a day. As weight-bearing strengthening exercises, toe raises, heel walks, and toe walks should be incorporated to regain strength and coordination. Toe curling exercises with paper or towel and marble picking should also be included for strengthening of the foot musculature table.

Table: Structured strength training progression.

1st set: 10 repetitions	2nd set: 10 repetitions	3rd set: 10 repetitions	4th set: 10 repetitions*
0 lbs (0 kg)	5 lbs (0.23 kg)	1 lbs (0.45 kg)	1.5 lbs (0.68 kg)
1(0.45)	1.5 (0.68)	2 (0.91)	3 (1.36)
2 (0.91)	3 (1.36)	4 (1.81)	5 (2.27)
3 (1.36)	4.5 (2.04)	6 (2.72)	8 (3.63)
4 (1.81)	6 (2.72)	8 (3.63)	10 (4.54)
5 (2.27)	7.5 (3.40)	10 (4.54)	15 (6.80)
7.5 (3.40)	11.25 (5.10)	15 (6.80)	20 (9.07)
10 (4.54)	15 (6.80)	20 (9.07)	25 (11.34)
12.5 (5.67)	18.75 (8.51)	25 (11.34)	30 (13.61)
15 (6.80)	22.5 (10.21)	30 (13.61)	35 (15.88)
17.5 (7.94)	26.25 (11.91)	35 (15.88)	40 (18.14)
20 (9.07)	30 (13.61)	40 (18.14)	45 (20.41)
22.5 (10.21)	33.75 (15.31)	45 (20.41)	50 (22.68)

25 (11.34)	37.5 (17.01)	50 (22.68)	55 (24.95)
27.5 (12.47)	41.25 (18.71)	55 (24.95)	60 (27.22)
30 (13.61)	45 (20.41)	60 (27.22)	65 (29.48)
32.5 (14.74)	48.75 (22.11)	65 (29.48)	70 (31.75)

The athlete should proceed to the next line when he/she can lock out (complete with correct form) the 4th set 10 times.

Improve Proprioception and Balance

Once the athlete achieves full weight-bearing without pain, proprioceptive training is started for the recovery of balance and postural control. Various devices have been designed for this phase of rehabilitation. Their use in performance with a series of progressive drills has effectively returned athletes to a high functional level. As somatosensory and visual feedback is altered, the athlete must develop consistent motor patterns even with inconsistent feedback. Furthermore, the athlete can be tested under various visual and support conditions. The simplest device for proprioceptive training is the wobble board. The athlete is instructed to stand on the wobble board on one foot and shift his or her weight, causing the disc's edge to scribe a continuous circular path. These exercises can be progressed by having the athlete use different-sized hemispheres and by varying visual input. A common progression when performing balance exercise is to move from a position of non-weight-bearing to weight-bearing, bilateral stance to unilateral stance, eyes open to eyes closed, firm surface to soft surface, uneven or moving surface. Another variant is when the therapist manually moves the ankle and foot through various positions and then asks the athlete to actively and passively replicate the joint angles. This helps improving joint position sense. As the body is trained to sense directions from perturbation, sensory input is received from all parts of the body and sent to the central nervous system via afferent pathways. Therefore, conscious and unconscious appreciation is important to protect functional joint stability. Proprioception is useful for preventing injury in slow, moderately quick, or even quick tasks; however, it may not be adequate for forces that challenge the neuromuscular system at the highest levels. The therapist should also focus on variability of speed and intensity while training proprioception and balance table.

Table: Proprioceptive exercises (the variation and changes should be according to the athlete's requirements).

No material	Ball	Balance board	Ball + balance board
Exercise 1: One-legged stance with the knee flexed. Step out on the other leg with the knee flexed, and keep balance for 5 s. Repeat 10 times for both legs. Variations 1 2 3 4	Exercise 3: *Make pairs. Both stand in one-legged stance with the knee flexed. Keep a distance of 5 m. Throw and catch a ball 5 times while maintaining balance. Repeat 10 times for both legs. Variations 1 2	Exercise 5: One legged stance on the balance board with the knee flexed. Maintain balance for 30 s and change stance leg. Repeat twice for both legs. Variations 1 2 3 4	Exercise 10: Athlete stands with both feet on the balance board. Throw and catch a ball 10 times with one hand while maintaining balance. Repeat twice.

Exercise 2: One-legged stance with the hip and the knee flexed. Step out on the other leg with the hip and knee flexed, and keep balance for 5 s. Repeat 10 times for both legs. Variations 1 2 3 4	Exercise 4: *Make pairs. Stand both in one-legged stance with the hip and knee flexed. Keep a distance of 5 m. Throw and catch a ball 5 times while maintaining balance. Repeat 10 times for both legs. Variations 1 2	Exercise 6: One-legged stance on the balance board with the hip and knee flexed. Maintain balance for 30 s and change stance leg. Repeat twice for both legs. Variations 1 2 3 4	Exercise 11: Athlete stands in one-legged stance with the knee flexed on the balance board. Throw and catch a ball 10 times with one hand while maintaining balance. Repeat twice for both legs. Variations 1 2
Variations on basic exercises: The standing leg is stretched. The standing leg is flexed. The standing is stretched and first eyes are opened, followed by eyes closed. The standing leg is flexed and first eyes are open followed by eyes closed. The standing leg is stretched and upper hand technique (throwing the ball from above the head). The standing leg is flexed and upper hand technique. The standing leg is stretched and lower hand technique (throwing the ball while keeping the hand below the waist). The standing leg is flexed and lower hand technique. *This can be done by the therapist, and the athlete or the athlete can stand opposite to the wall at a distance of 5 m.		Exercise 7: Step slowly over the balance board with one foot on the balance board. Maintain the balance board in a horizontal position while stepping over. Repeat 10 times for both legs.	Exercise 12: Athlete stands in one-legged stance with the hip and knee flexed on the balance board; the other has the same position on the floor. Throw and/or catch a ball 10 times with one hand while maintaining balance. Repeat twice for both legs Variations 1 2
		Exercise 8: Stand with both feet on the balance board. Make 10 knee flexions while maintaining balance.	Exercise 13: Athlete stands with both feet on the balance board. Throw the ball with an upper hand technique 10 times while maintaining balance. Repeat twice for both legs. Variations 5 6 7 8
		Exercise 9: One-legged stance on the balance board with the knee flexed. Make 10 knee flexions while maintaining balance. Repeat twice for both legs.	Exercise 14: Athlete stands in one-legged stance with the knee flexed on the balance board. Throw the ball with an upper hand technique 10 times while maintaining balance. Repeat twice for both legs. Variations 5 6 7 8

*All the exercises done by the Athlete, can be done in pairs or the athlete can stand opposite to a wall at distance of 5 m.

Sports-specific Training

Once the distance walked by the athlete is no longer limited by pain, he/she can be put on sports-specific training or advanced training. The use of sports-specific means of training, parallel to general conditioning training, leads to considerable improvement of performance among athletes. The sports-specific training includes intricate activities like jogging which eventually progresses to running, backward running, and pattern running. Circles and figure of 8 are commonly employed patterns. These activities can also be done using ankle weight to increase the difficulty level. Star excursion balance training can also be used in which the athlete stands on the sprained ankle while using another foot to reach as far as possible in eight directions as outlined in the Star Excursion Balance Test. The exercise can consist of 8–10 rounds clockwise and counterclockwise foot reach with 3 s rest between each direction. The difficulty level can be increased by adding variations to the exercise such as with the sprained ankle (affected leg's knee) flexed, eyes opened, followed by eyes closed. At higher speed, i.e., at an angular velocity of 120°/s, the eversion to inversion ratio is >1.0, adding to the risk of injuries. Hence, resistance bands can be used to strengthen the ankle musculature, i.e., training an athlete on an isokinetic machine while tying the band on the affected ankle and with the therapist holding the other end and maintaining the resistance through the movement. This should be done for 15–20 repetitions 1–2 times/day and with increasing progression. Specific training can include functional activities on various surfaces, e.g., trampoline and foam, and in water with weights. Repetitions should be 5–20, 1–2 times/day.

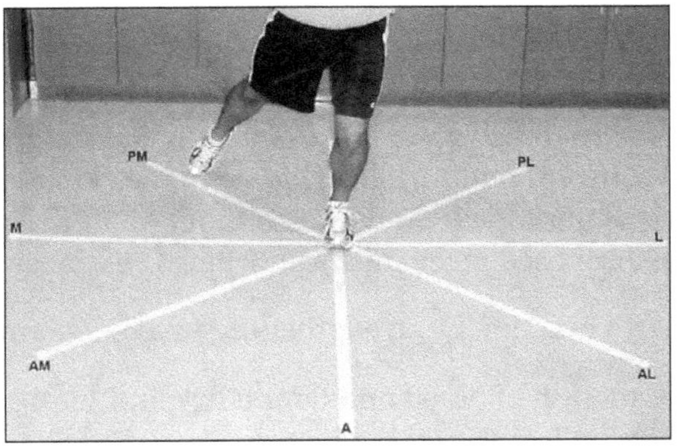

Star excursion balance test. Note: Star Excursion Balance Test for left-leg dominant participants (Posterior direction is behind athlete's right leg). Abbreviations: A, anterior; AM, anterior-medial; M, medial; PM, posterior-medial; P, posterior; PL, posterior-lateral; L, lateral; AL, anterior-lateral.

Criteria for return to Sports

The athlete can participate fully in the sporting activity once the pain has been reduced completely. The progression should be gradual in order to stress the ligaments without causing further harm. Full participation should be allowed once the athlete has complete range of motion, 80–90% of preinjury strength and a normal gait pattern including the ability to perform sports-specific activities such as cutting and landing without any compensation due to the injury. The athlete should be able to complete a full practice without pain or swelling.

Taping and Bracing

Taping and bracing the ankle can be used for prevention as well as for rehabilitation. Application of tapes and braces is helpful in the prevention of lateral ankle sprains and in the recurrence of injuries. Application of a tape or a brace increases the afferent feedback from cutaneous receptors, which lead to improved ankle joint position sense.

This increased stimulation results in a more appropriate positioning of the unstable ankle and protects it from re-injury. Hence it helps improve joint position sense through proprioceptive mechanism.

Taping: The major role of taping is to prevent extreme range of movements and to reduce abnormal patterns of movements of the ankle. Various techniques are in use, but the most common techniques are basket weave with stirrup and heel lock and basket weave and heel lock techniques. Taping has mechanical effects: it decreases movement of inversion and plantar flexion and increases the force required for a specific displacement in inversion and plantar flexion. Taping helps in decreasing the extent of non-weight-bearing talar tilt. It also limits the full weight-bearing talar tilt. Athletes with the greatest instability benefit most from the tape. Although taping does improve mechanical instability, the restricting effect is lost after varying periods of exercise. About 40% of taping effect is lost after 10 min of vigorous exercise like jumping, pivoting, running, etc.

Kinesio taping: Unlike structurally supportive tape, such as white athletic tape, Kinesio tape is therapeutic in nature. It differs from the traditional athletic tape with respect to its elasticity, i.e., it can be stretched up to 140% of its original length before applying it on the skin. It provides a constant pulling (shear) force to the skin unlike traditional white athletic tape. The fabric of this tape is air permeable and water resistant and can be worn for repetitive days. The proposed mechanisms in which the Kinesio tape works are:

- It corrects muscle function by strengthening weakened muscles.
- It improves circulation of blood and lymph by eliminating tissue fluid or bleeding beneath the skin by moving the muscle.
- It reduces pain through neurological suppression.
- It repositions subluxated joints by relieving abnormal muscle tension, helping to return the function of fascia and muscles.
- It improves proprioception through increased stimulation to cutaneous mechanoreceptors.

Bracing: Ankle bracing can make a significant contribution to preventing lateral ankle sprains. It also shows a significant reduction in the frequency of ankle sprain recurrence. Ankle braces have certain advantages over tape allowing self-application without the expertise of qualified personnel. They are convenient to apply and to remove; they are reusable, readjustable, and washable. There are nonrigid and semirigid braces. The nonrigid ones are often made of canvas or a neoprene-type material, which can easily be slipped on and off, and some are with additional lacing. The semirigid braces mostly consist of bimalleolar struts made of thermoplastic materials attached by Velcro straps. Nowadays different braces are used such as lace-up braces and the Swede-O (Swede-O-Universal, North Branch, MN) and multiple models by McDavid Sports Medical Products (Woodridge, IL); lace-up braces with straps such as the ASO

(Medical Specialties, Charlotte, NC), the RocketSoc (DonJoy Orthopedics, Inc., Vista, CA), and the Ankle Brace Lock (Breg, Vista, CA); and semirigid plastic braces with strapping configurations such as the Ankle Ligament Protector (DonJoy Orthopedics, Inc.), the Universal Ankle Stirrup (DonJoy Orthopedics, Inc.), the T2 Active Ankle Support (Active Ankle, Louisville, KY) and the Ultra Ankle, and the Guardian Ankle (McDavid Sports Medical Products).

Semirigid brace like Swede-O-Universal and nonrigid brace like subtalar supports provide a better non-weight-bearing restriction in plantar flexion, dorsiflexion, and eversion than taping after 15 min of activity. A strong thermoplastic semirigid ankle brace significantly reduces talar and subtalar motions of plantarflexion, inversion, and adduction. In summary, ankle taping and bracing:

- Restrict ankle range of motion.
- Reduce injury and recurrence rate.
- Improve proprioception.
- Lose limitation of movement after exercise.
- Have no negative effect on most performance tests.
- Have little negative effect on other joints.

Grade III Lateral Ankle Sprains

Grade III lateral ankle sprains occur when there is a complete rupture of both ATFL and CFL. Although the initial line of management remains a functional rehabilitation, surgery should be considered if the symptoms persist. The feeling of giving way, defined as functional instability or true mechanical instability, is frequently experienced. This can be demonstrated by provocative tests such as the anterior drawer or talar tilt (either clinically or by stress radiography). Particular attention should be directed at the diagnosis and correction of subtle subtalar instability in individuals with functional instability. Surgical repairs are aimed at the reconstruction of the normal anatomy by overlapping the existing joint capsule and lateral ligaments. The rehabilitation protocol post-surgery remains the same as that of the conservative treatment.

Hamstring Strain

A hamstring strain or 'pulled hamstring' is a tear to one of the hamstring muscles. Sudden sharp pain is felt at the back of the thigh which can range from mild to severe.

Hamstring Strain Symptoms

Symptoms of a hamstring strain usually consist of a sudden sharp pain at the back of the thigh, either whilst sprinting or performing a fast stretching movement such as a high kick. Hamstring strains are graded 1, 2 or 3 depending on how bad they are.

- A grade 1 hamstring strain is relatively mild. You may feel a twinge or tightness at the time of injury, with little or no swelling.
- A grade 2 is more severe.
- If you have a grade 2 strain you will feel a sudden sharp pain at the time of injury. Swelling is likely and you will be unable to continue playing or training.

Other Injuries causing Posterior Thigh Pain

- Cramp.
- Hamstring tendon strain.
- Femur stress fracture.

What is a Pulled Hamstring?

A hamstring strain (pulled hamstring) is a tear to any one or more of the hamstring muscles at the back of the thigh.

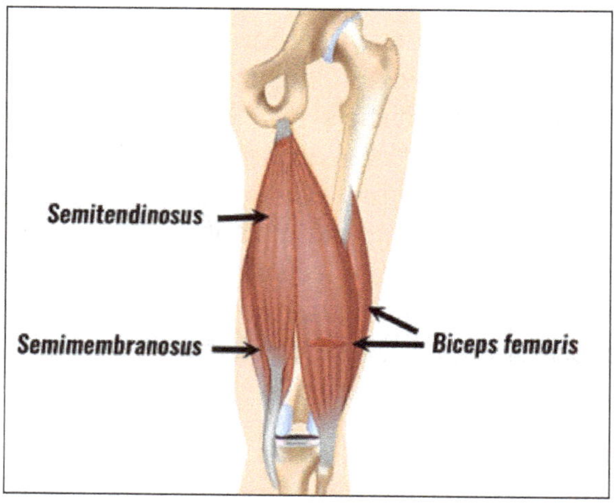

The Hamstring muscle group consists of three separate muscles:

- Semitendinosus.
- Semimembranosus.
- Biceps femoris.

The muscles originate from the lower part of the pelvic bone (ischial tuberosity) and insert into the back of the shin bone (tibia). When they contract, they bend (flex) the knee and help extend the hip (move the leg backwards).

What Causes a Hamstring Strain?

Hamstring strains usually occur in two different ways. They are either sprinting related or stretch related for example in martial arts, gymnastics or dancing.

Sprint Related Hamstring Strains

- During sprinting the hamstring muscles work extremely hard. In particular, at a point just before the foot strikes the ground they decelerate the tibia (shin) very quickly. It is at this point that the hamstring is most likely to tear.
- Sprint related hamstring injuries usually occur lower down the biceps femoris muscle. More specifically, where the muscle joins to the tendon. They often feel worse initially, but recover more quickly.

Stretch Related Hamstring Strains

- Stretch related injuries usually occur higher up at the back of the thigh. Most commonly the in the tendon of the semimembranosus muscle.
- These injuries may take longer to heal because the blood supply to the tendon is not as good.

Referred Pain

- Referred pain is caused by problems elsewhere such as the lower back and hip, but is felt at the back of the leg.
- These may increase the likelihood of suffering a hamstring strain and should always be considered, particularly if you suffer from recurrent hamstring strains.

Hamstring Strain Treatment and Rehabilitation

Treatment is divided into immediate first aid, then longer-term treatment which begins after the initial acute stage of healing.

Immediate First Aid

The acute phase of hamstring strain rehabilitation usually lasts 3 to 4 days depending on how bad your injury is. Complete rest is advised, with no running or playing active sport allowed and as little walking as possible. Apply the PRICE principles of protection, rest, ice, compression, and elevation.

- Protection: Protect your muscle from further injury. This means leaving the field of play or stopping exercise as soon as possible.
- Rest: From anything that causes pain, both immediately after injury and longer term whilst your muscle strain is healing.
- Ice: Apply cold therapy for 15 minutes every hour in the early stages, or at least 3 or 4 times per day. Ice should not be applied directly to the skin as it may cause ice burns. Instead, wrap in a wet tea towel. Commercially available cold packs and wraps that are just as effective.
- Compression: Use a compression bandage or thigh support to apply compression. This can be worn all the time during the acute stage to help reduce swelling and support the muscle.
- Elevation: Elevate the limb as much as you can because this will help swelling and tissue fluids drain away.

Once the initial acute phase has passed you move into the sub-acute phase.

Sports Massage

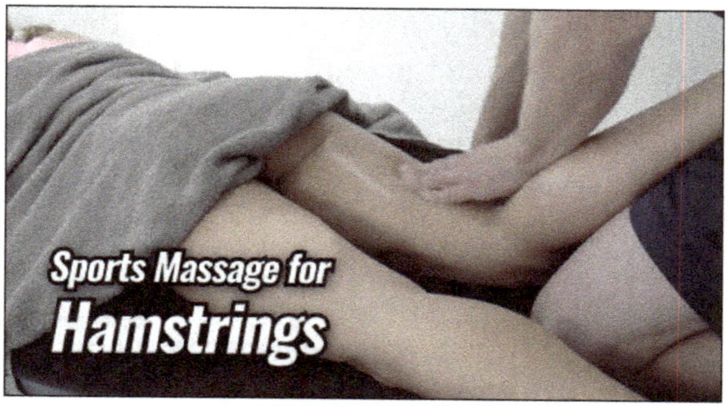

Sports Massage or soft tissue massage can be used at this stage but the pressure must be very light and superficial, to begin with, but can gradually get deeper as the days/weeks pass.

Massage can help to break down any scar tissue that has formed and can help to relax tight muscles and stimulate blood flow to the area and all of this aids the healing process and may increase flexibility. Light massage can be applied daily initially but later on, as the techniques become deeper, more recovery time between sessions may be required.

Hamstring Strain Exercises

Both stretching and strengthening exercises are important. After the initial acute stage, very gentle static stretching exercises can begin as long as they are pain-free. As your injury heals, dynamic stretching which involves movement is introduced and eventually sports-specific drills.

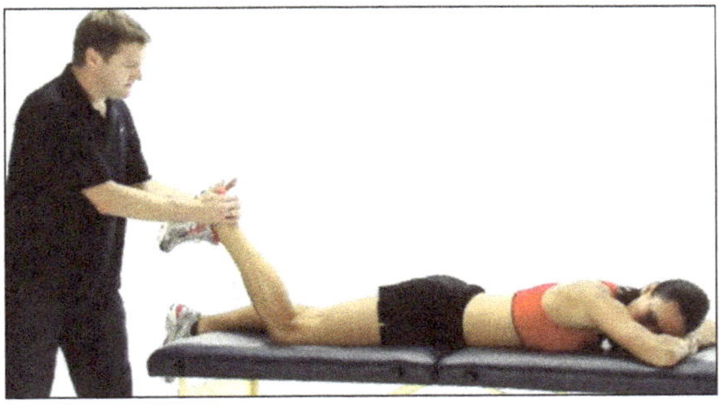

Hamstring Kinesiology Taping

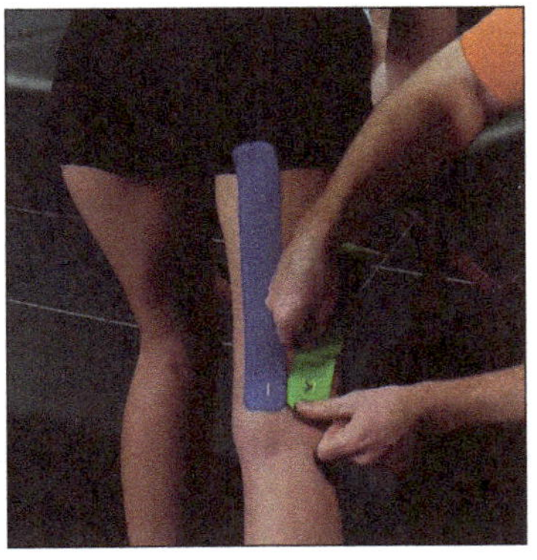

Kinesiology taping can be applied during the later stages of rehabilitation by encouraging activation of the muscle fibres.

Hamstring Strain Exercises

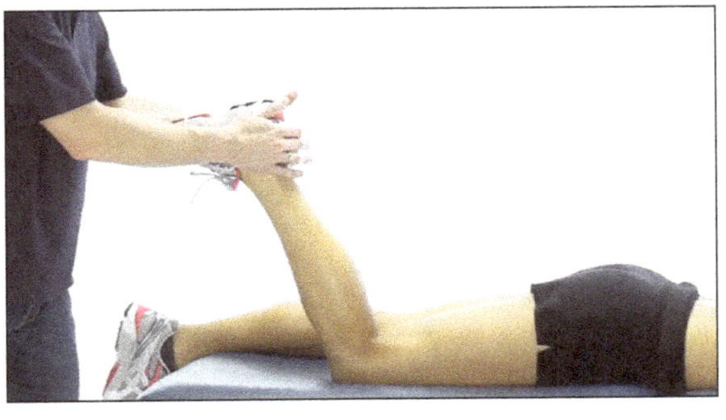

Both stretching and strengthening exercises are important. After the initial acute stage, very gentle static stretching exercises can begin as long as they are pain-free. As your injury heals, dynamic stretching which involves movement is introduced and eventually sports-specific drills.

Strengthening exercises also begin gently with isometric contractions and progress through to advanced hamstring exercises.

Plantar Fasciitis

Plantar fasciitis is probably the most common cause of pain under the heel. Often a combination of approaches is needed to cure this stubborn injury.

Plantar Fasciitis Symptoms

- Pain under the heel which develops gradually over time.
- Often pain may radiate forwards into the arch of the foot.
- There may be tenderness in the sole of the foot and under the heel when pressing in. This can range from being slightly uncomfortable to acutely painful.
- Pain is usually worse first thing in the morning and improves during the day.

Assessment Tests

A professional therapist would undertake a full assessment. This may include:

- Case history.
- Physical examination.
- Biomechanical analysis.
- They may use X-rays or other imaging techniques to diagnose plantar fasciitis.

Other heel injuries, particularly bruised heel can have similar symptoms. Below we outline some common differences between plantar fasciitis and bruised heel.

Table: Planter Fasiitis vs. Bruised heel.

Sign or symptom	Plantar fasciitis	Bruised heel
Do you have pain under the heel	✓	✓
Has the pain occurred gradually?	✓	✓
Is pain worse first thing in the morning?	✓	×
Is pain worse trying to walk after a period of rest?	✓	×
Does the pain ease off only to return later?	✓	×
Is the pain directly under the heel?	✓	✓
Does pain radiate into the arch?	✓	×

Is it painful when pressing in under the heel?	✓	✓
Is it painful pressing into the arch of the foot?	✓	×
Do you have flat feet or overpronate?	✓	×
Do you have tight calf muscles?	✓	×

Plantar Fasciitis Causes and Anatomy

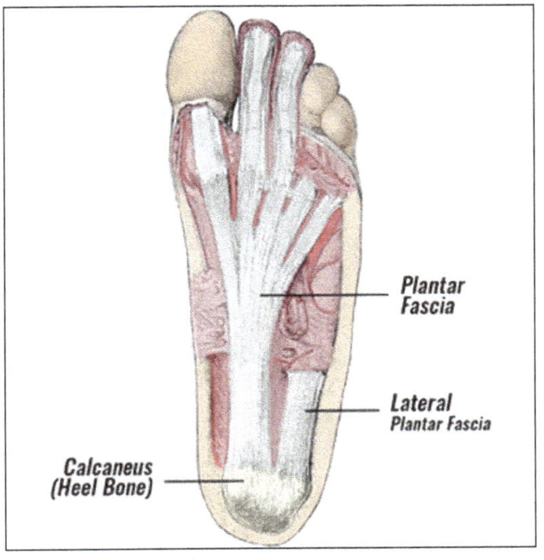

The Plantar Fascia (or plantar aponeurosis) is a broad, thick band of tissue which runs from under the heel bone (calcaneus), to the front of the foot. Its function is to provide support to the foot when standing and shock absorption when running. Inflammation or degeneration of the tendon where the fascia originates at the heel causes pain.

Heel Spurs

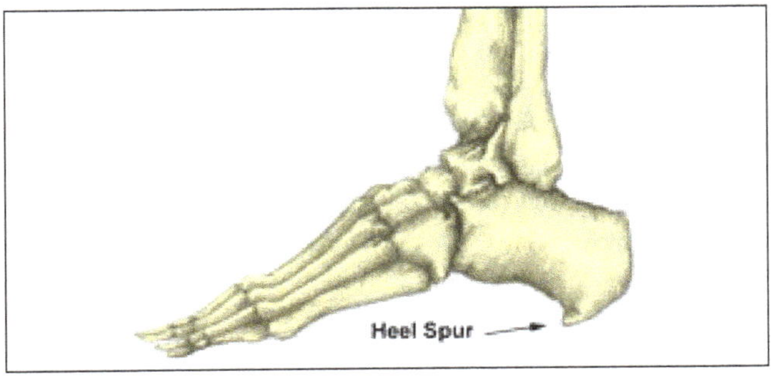

Sometimes a bony growth, known as a heel spur develops at the point where the fascia attaches to the heel. But not all cases of plantar fasciitis have a heel spur, and many heel spurs have no symptoms.

Plantar Fasciitis or Plantar Fasciopathy?

The term Plantar fasciitis refers to inflammation ('itis' means inflammation). Traditionally people thought inflammation was the issue. However, studies have shown actual inflammatory cells are not present in most cases. Therefore, degeneration of the tissues is thought to be a more likely cause. Hence the term Plantar fasciopathy is more appropriate.

Causes of Plantar Fasciitis

Overuse is thought to be the main cause of plantar fasciitis. It is more common in sports which involve running, dancing or jumping. However, there are a number of factors which can increase your chances of developing Plantar fasciitis heel pain:

Foot Biomechanics

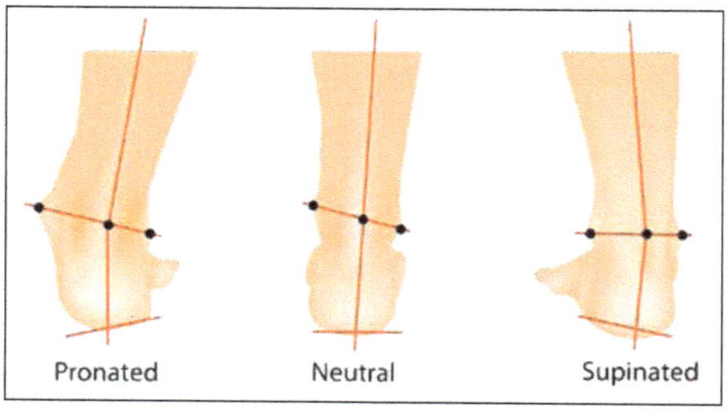

Overpronation is where the foot rolls in or flattens too much when running or walking. As the foot flattens, it stretches the plantar fascia more than normal, therefore increasing the strain on the tissues.

A foot which has a high arch is known as pes cavus. This foot type is often rigid and therefore unable to absorb shock and impact forces. Therefore, the strain on the plantar fascia is increased.

Footwear

Wearing inappropriate footwear such as very flat and unsupporting shoes can increase the likelihood of developing plantar fasciitis. If you are a runner then choosing the correct running shoes for your foot type is essential. If you overpronated then a motion control shoe is best. Oversupinators often have a high arch and a neutral shoe with cushioning is usually advised.

Bodyweight

Overweight individuals or those who do a lot of heaving lifting at the workplace increased loads on the foot. Therefore, increasing the chances of developing heel pain.

Flexibility

If you have tight calf muscles or plantar fascia then you are at a higher risk of developing plantar fasciitis. Or, if you have tight hamstrings or gluteal muscles then this also increases your risk because of the effect they have on foot biomechanics.

Plantar Fasciitis Treatment

Treatment consists of reducing pain and inflammation, stretching the plantar fascia and lower leg muscles and identifying potential causes.

A gradual return to fitness is important. Heel pain can be very stubborn to treat and often a combination of approaches is best in treating plantar fasciitis.

Self-help Treatment

- Applying the PRICE principles of protection, rest, ice, compression and elevation to relieve pain and inflammation. Apply ice or a cold therapy wrap. Do not apply ice directly to the skin as it may cause ice burns. Wrap ice in a wet tea towel or use a commercially available gel pack.
- Apply ice or cold therapy for up to 10 minutes every hour whilst it is particularly painful. Reduce this to 3 times a day as symptoms improve.

Plantar Fasciitis Taping

Plantar fasciitis taping is an excellent way of instantly relieving symptoms. It works by supporting the arch of the foot and reducing the strain on the plantar fascia. This, therefore, allows the tissues to heal. You may need to apply tape regularly until symptoms resolve but many people notice an immediate improvement.

Protect and support the foot by wearing comfortable shoes or trainers. Hard or flat-soled shoes are likely to make symptoms worse. You can wear a cushioning heel pad or insole to help relieve pain. However, if over pronation is an issue then orthotic type insoles will be more appropriate long term.

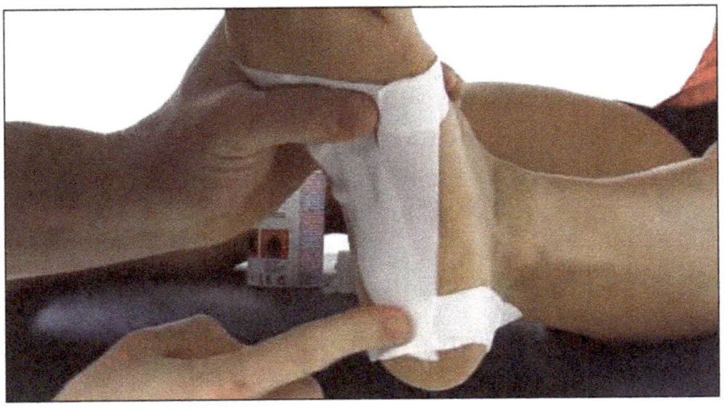

Plantar Fasciitis Night Splint

Stretching exercises can begin as soon as pain allows. A plantar fasciitis night splint is a very effective way of stretching the plantar fascia under the heel. You wear the splint overnight, or as long as you can until it becomes too painful. Gradually you should be able to wear it for longer because it helps prevent the fascia tightening overnight.

What can a Professional Do?

- A professional therapist can make an accurate diagnosis and advise on a full treatment and rehabilitation plan.
- A doctor may prescribe anti-inflammatory medication such as ibuprofen. This may be effective in the early stages to reduce pain and inflammation. But long term use may actually inhibit healing.
- The therapist may use electrotherapy such as ultrasound or laser treatment to reduce pain and inflammation.

Massage for Plantar Fasciitis

In the later stages, a professional therapist may apply deep tissue massage to help stretch and relax the plantar fascia.

They may also use gait analysis to identify any biomechanical issues and prescribe orthotic inserts. These help control the position of the heel, reducing overpronation and therefore the strain on the foot.

For more stubborn injuries a doctor may use a corticosteroid injection. Platelet-rich plasma injections have also been shown to be effective. If symptoms do not resolve then surgery is an option but this is rare.

Plantar Fasciitis Surgery

Surgery is used in around 5% of people whose symptoms do not improve after a minimum of nine months, even after continuous treatment. However, the success rate is still only estimated at around 70-80%. In most cases now, a procedure called a plantar fascia release is performed. This releases (cuts) between 30 and 50% of the fascia's fibers. This helps to reduce the stress on the fascia. Complications can include nerve damage, fallen arches, infection and ongoing symptoms. Recovery after surgery if successful is around 9 to 12 weeks before the patient may return to work.

Plantar Fasciitis Exercises

Exercises to stretch the plantar fascia and the calf muscles are important. Resting alone may reduce pain and inflammation but if part of the cause is tension in fascia then the injury is likely to recur.

Plantar Fascia Stretch

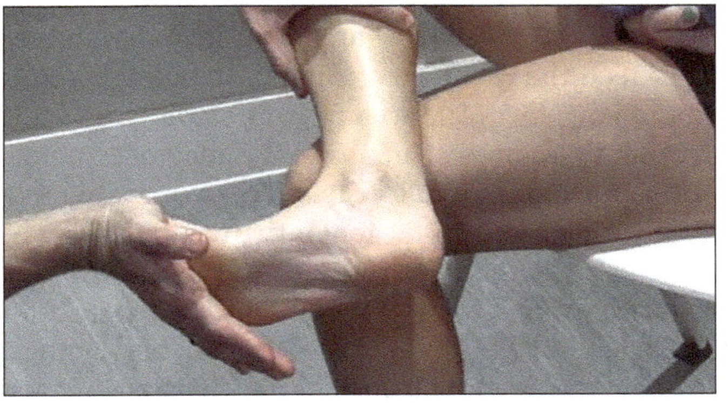

The plantar fascia stretch is done by pulling the foot and toes upwards aiming to feel a stretch in the arch of the foot. Rolling the foot over a ball can also help stretch underneath the foot.

Calf Muscle Stretches

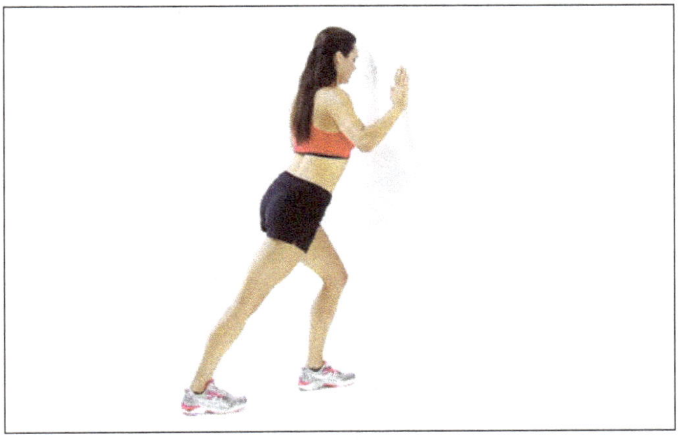

Calf stretches with the leg straight (to target the larger gastrocnemius muscle) and with the knee bent (targeting the lower soleus muscles) can be done 3 to 5 times a day. Hold stretches for up to 30 seconds at a time and they should be done pain-free.

Strengthening exercises are not normally needed, however scrunching a towel up with the toes can get the small muscles of the foot working.

Meniscus Tear

The knee joint is the largest and most complicated joint in the human body. Bone structures, capsules, menisci, and ligaments provide static stability in the knee joint and are responsible for dynamic stabilization of the muscles and tendons. Menisci are fibrocartilage structures that cover two-thirds of the tibial plateau joint surface. The main functions of the meniscus are load sharing and loading of the tibiofemoral joint, shock absorption, helping to feed the cartilage by facilitating dissociation of the joint fluid, and contributing to the joint fit by increasing joint stability and joint contact surface area. Menisci are frequently injured structures. The incidence of acute meniscal tears is 60 per 100,000. It is more common in males. Trauma-related tears are common in patients under 30 years of age, whereas degenerative complex tears increase in patients over 30 years of age. There may not be a significant trauma story, especially in degenerative meniscus tears. They are sports traumas that come to the fore in the etiology of meniscus tears. It is the football that has the greatest risk of creating a meniscus lesion, followed by athletics, American football, and skiing. There is an indication for repair in peripheral ruptures where blood flow is excessive. In the central rupture where blood is not present, the treatment is meniscectomy.

The knee is an open joint to frequent injuries in sports activities. Direct impacts, forced movements, or repetitive overloads can cause anatomical damage. Menisci are formed from fibrous cartilage. It has a shock-absorbing feature. The main tasks are providing load transfer, increasing joint surface contact area and joint stability, and contributing to proprioception. A total of 100,000 people per year are found to have meniscus rupture in 60–70. The most common pathology associated with meniscal tears is anterior cruciate ligament (ACL) ruptures.

Today, in addition to professional sportsmen, people participate in sports activities for hobby purposes. Increasing interest in sports with high risk of injury, such as skiing, snowboarding, and mountain biking, has increased the frequency of traumatic meniscal tear. Decision-making process is difficult in professional sportsmen. Approximately 40% of all sports injuries involve the knee joint. Meniscus injuries account for 14.5% of these injuries. The most risky period in terms of age is between the ages of 20 and 29. Male to female ratio of meniscus proplemia in sports injuries is 2–4/1. The medial-lateral meniscus injury rate for all age groups was reported as 3/1. However, lateral meniscus tears are more common in young professional athletes. According to the age distribution, the medial meniscus tear is more likely to occur in the athletes who are under 30 years old and laterally in sportsmen over 30 years. In an epidemiological study of National Basketball Association (NBA) basketball players, 87.8% of meniscal tears are isolated, and 12.2% are associated with ligament injuries, often ACL. Acute ACL injuries are more common in lateral meniscus, and chronic ACL injuries are more common in medial meniscus tears. Body mass index (BMI) is specified in professional basketball players as a risk factor. It has been reported that especially above 25, it increases the risk of rupture more in the lateral meniscus. The high physical activity during play was more associated with the lateral meniscus. In an epidemiological study of athletic knee injuries, the distribution of 836 medial meniscus injuries according to sports branches was examined. Soccer was 32.7%, skiing 22.4%, tennis 7.8%, handball

5.4%, and cycling 3.5%. In the distribution of 284 lateral meniscus injuries, 34.5% of football, 19% of skiing, 9.8% of handball, 6.6% of tennis, and 3.5% of cycling sources were stated. In gymnastics and dancers doing lateral, tennis, and jogging, the risk of medial meniscus injuries is greater. Most of the injuries occur during the competition and are thought to be caused by faulty warming or overloading. 10–19 years is the period when lateral meniscus injuries are seen in sportsmen at the second frequency. It is thought that rapid and variable physiology of the age of growth has increased meniscus injuries in this age group. Nowadays, with the understanding of biomechanics and functions of the meniscus, tissue preservation has become the mainstay of treatment. Exposure to high physical activity levels and relatively early age causes injury to the athletes in terms of degenerative arthrosis.

The diagnosis of symptomatic meniscus rupture can be made during the anatomy of the patient. The common complaints of patients are pain during hanging and flexion, which starts after the knee swelling or excessive flexion. On physical examination, joint tenderness, McMurray test, and Apley test were described as the most commonly used tests. Magnetic resonance imaging (MRI) can diagnose approximately 95% of cases. Because non-symptomatic individuals can also detect meniscal tears with MRI, treatment decisions should be made by combining them with the clinical findings of the patient, not just the MRI outcome. Many features should be taken into account when deciding on surgical treatment of meniscus tears. Among the factors that are effective in deciding on surgical technique for menisci are patient complaints, age, rupture size, and additional pathologies associated with morphology.

Total meniscectomy has been used extensively in the pre-arthroscopic era and has caused many athletes to lose their sporting life. It has been shown that partial meniscectomy causes irreversible damage to joint cartilage in the long term. Since the 1980s, the development of arthroscopic techniques and the ability to repair the menstrual blood, and thus the healing possibilities, have led to the repair of suitable tears. Longitudinal tears, usually in the peripheral 25% area, are suitable for repairs in young and sporty people. With the understanding that menisci are indispensable for knee health today, indications for repair especially in lateral meniscus tears have been expanded.

In the beginning, conventional sewing techniques have been described as repairs from the inside to the outside and from the outside. With a variety of meniscal fixators (meniscus fixation materials), the possibility of vascular nerve injury with complete internal repair has been reduced, and operation times have been shortened.

In comparison with biomechanical stitches, conventional stitches have shown remarkably superior durability than meniscal fixators in many studies.

When performing arthroscopic surgery, care should first be taken to protect the meniscus tissue. Accompanying lesions should be evaluated carefully, especially with frequent ACL problems. All problems should be solved together by following a holistic approach in treatment. These injuries cause serious morbidity in the short term when not properly treated. In the long term, it may also lead to degenerative changes in the knee joint resulting in osteoarthritis.

Therefore, the treatment of meniscus injuries is very important. Today, it is understood that meniscus is protected as much as possible. Current treatment methods are being implemented and developed on the basis of this principle.

Meniscus Tear

Meniscus tears are the result of traumatic, degenerative, or congenital pathologies. Loads exceeding the normal endurance limit may result in a tear. In degenerative menisci, ruptures may also occur at normal loads. Traumatic tears usually occur in active people, aged between 10 and 40 years. Degenerative tears are generally over 40 years of age. Such tears are often associated with other degenerative changes in the cartilage and bone tissues of the knee.

Management of Treatment

Accelerating degenerative changes in the meniscus-deficient knees and the menisci played a key role in the functioning of the meniscus leading us to focus on the protection of the meniscus. In early 1948, Fairbank showed that total meniscectomy accelerated the radiological change in the knee. This was changed by partial meniscectomy.

There is no randomized controlled trial showing that arthroscopic meniscus repair has a long-term benefit for joint protection. However, good results to date suggest that this may reduce the incidence of early degenerative changes.

All meniscus tears would not cause clinical symptoms. It has been shown that the tibial asymptomatic meniscus tears, which are intact and have biomechanical function, can recover spontaneously.

The results of not treating meniscus tears are not very clear. Experimental animal studies have shown that meniscal tears may result in chondropathy and osteoarthritis.

Clinical studies could not explain whether meniscal injury or articular cartilage damage developed first. A recent study by Christoforakis evaluated 497 consecutive knee arthroscopies in patients with meniscal tear. These complex and horizontal tears were found to be statistically increased in outerbridge grade III or IV joint cartilage damage. Moreover, complex and horizontal tears had excessive joint damage compared to other types of tears. Nevertheless, the result does not answer which of the meniscus tears or articular degeneration occurred first.

The general approach is to actively tear the young patients with clinical and radiological examinations including X-ray and MRI. If there is a tear or is very suspicious, arthroscopy and meniscus protection surgery are recommended. Non-operative treatment option is used in patients with suspected degenerative tears. The debridement of the degenerated meniscus is well documented that it cannot always result in long-term relief.

Non-operative Treatment

Small peripheral tears in young patients can be treated without surgery. The difficulty is to decide whether the tear is stable or not. Weiss et al. retrospectively reviewed 3612 arthroscopic procedures for meniscus lesions. They found 80 (2.2%) meniscus tears which were considered stable. They were not treated. Six patients presented for arthroscopy again due to meniscus symptoms.

Physiotherapy has been shown to be beneficial to patients with degenerative meniscus tears. In a recent published randomized control study, patients who underwent surgical debridement with physiotherapy showed no better results than those who received only physiotherapy.

Some patients with degenerative meniscal tears recover after a single corticosteroid injection into the knee. Corticosteroids are the first-line treatment for degenerative meniscus in the absence of locking symptoms.

Because of the high functional expectations and the need for early return to sports, it is still preferred in selected cases.

In the red-red zone, stable, incomplete longitudinal tears with a size below 1 cm may be suitable for conservative treatment. Bucket handle, radial, parrot beak, oblique tears, and degenerative and complex tears are not suitable for conservative methods. Conservative treatment can be used as a temporary treatment method in athletes, who are frequently asymptomatic in the season.

Selection should be made when deciding on conservative treatment. Abnormal stresses should be avoided in the early period of rupture. The development of cartilage lesions after aggressive rehabilitation of a young professional athlete with lateral meniscus radial rupture to return to early sports shows that this treatment is not innocent. It should be kept in mind that meniscus tears, which cannot be repaired, may cause cartilage lesions due to mechanical problems that occur even if they are not symptomatic in athletes. Surgical treatment should be prioritized especially in athletes.

Operative Management

Total Meniscectomy

With the development of arthroscopic techniques and understanding of biomechanics, the importance of meniscus has increased. Treatment led to a shift toward the protection of the meniscus tissue. Total meniscectomy treatment is rarely practiced today.

Open Repair

It was one of the first ways to repair meniscus tears. It is now used to fix the meniscus as part of the management of tibial plateau fractures.

Arthroscopic Repair

The high expectations and career concerns of the athletes have made the meniscus repairs even more important. Red-red zone often provides successful repairs due to the potential for cannulation. Discussions on repairs to the red-white zone are still ongoing. Midterm and long-term acceptable results after repair of red-white zone tears of 22 athletes are promising.

When deciding on the repair of meniscus in professional athletes, it is necessary to take into account the possibility of the meniscus recovery and to target 90% success. Considering the possible risks, the athletes should be careful to repair the tears in the red-white zone. White-white zone is considered to be the indication of repair today. But athletes should not consider arthroscopic repair.

Meniscus tear is present in 60% of ACL-ruptured patients. When the ligament is not repaired, the meniscus is becoming more complicated as it is not healed. For this reason, repairs should be done in the early period and in the same session.

Although it is accepted that there is an improvement in the repair area in about 6–8 weeks, the process actually lasts longer, and the athletes cannot return to competitive activities before 3 months. The improvement in the repaired meniscus depends on two basic elements. The first one is the extrinsic blood circulation, and the other is the ability to repair synovial fluid and fibrocartilage intrinsically. Histological studies after meniscus repair are based on animal experiments and cannot be fully adapted to human meniscus repair process. Therefore, the relationship between healing in tissue and return to movement is mostly based on clinical observations.

The success rates after repair vary. Pujol et al. reported success rates between 5 and 43% of meniscus repair in basketball players. According to Stein et al. in the 8-year follow-up, the rate of return to pre-traumatic activity in the group undergoing athletes was found to be 96.2%, and in the meniscectomy group, it was 50%. Paxton et al. found failure after meniscectomy was 3.7% and in repair group 20.7%.

It is reported that repair is better characterized by better functional scores and lower failure rates in the current meta-analysis of meniscectomy and repair. Reoperation depends not only on the technique but on the skill of the orthopedist, the tear itself, the age of the athlete, the level of activity, and the rehabilitation program applied. Evaluating the results of repair in athletes, failure in the medial meniscus was reported as 36.4%, and failure in the lateral meniscus was reported to be 5.6%.

Reoperation rates are high in medial meniscus repairs. This is due to the less mobility of the medial meniscus and to the greater load on the medial compartment. Late repair of medial tears has also been implicated as the cause of this failure.

Forty-two elite athletes and meniscus repair agressively recommend the study, after the repair reported 24% failure. Of the cases, 67% had medial meniscus, and 33% had lateral meniscus tears and a mean follow-up of 8.5 years.

The success of repair in the complete radial tears of the lateral meniscus is low. However, in the studies of Haklar et al., successful results are obtained in approximately half of the patients, and return to sports is provided. Nevertheless, these patients should be shared with the athlete who may be a candidate for meniscus transplant in the future.

The surgeon must also make efforts to repair the medial or lateral meniscus radial root tears in athletes. If the circumferential fibers are completely ruptured when the repair is not performed, the meniscus becomes functional. Therefore, primary repair of complete radial tears should be the first aim, especially in young athletes.

Radial tears in the posterior meniscus posterior are more promising because of the region's blood supply.

Failure to achieve successful results with today's repair techniques leads to new searches. The success of repair in meniscus tears combined with ACL reconstruction is thought to be the effect of growth factors and multipotent cells from the bone marrow. Similarly, synovial abrasion, trephination, mechanical stimulation, fibrin clot, or platelet-rich plasma (PRP) applications are always aimed for the same purpose.

The growth factors released after mechanical stimulation and trephination contribute positively to meniscus healing. Ochi et al. showed that the mediators increased to the highest level in the joint after 14 days of mechanical stimulation.

Trephination can be used successfully in the complete tears of the lateral meniscus posterior or in complete longitudinal tears less than 1 cm. Successful results of vertical, peripheral, and non-degenerative tears in trephination are seen in the literature.

In a recent study on the effect of PRP on meniscus repairs, no significant difference was found in functional scores. Rights et al. used microfracture to create an effect similar to ACL reconstruction, and this would also contribute positively to recovery in the repair area of multipotent cells.

Studies have shown that smoking has a negative effect on the results of meniscus repair.

For successful results, it is important to remember the importance of combining vertical mattress sutures from the inside to the outside as far as possible, with the microfracture method.

The presence of opposing views in the literature shows that there is still no consensus on rehabilitation and return to sports after repair. In the conservative approach, the return to sports takes a long period such as 3–6 months, while the aggressive approach is as short as 10 weeks. While limited conservative rehabilitation is recommended initially until the meniscus is healed, recent biomechanical studies report that early burden is not inconvenient. Even in animal experiments, it has been shown that blood flow to the repair site increases with mobilization.

In a randomized controlled trial by Lind et al., the functional scores with MRI and arthroscopy are evaluated. The rate of failure was found to be 28% in the limited rehabilitation group and 36% in the nonrestricted rehabilitation group.

As a result, we can say that the trend toward accelerated rehabilitation in the current studies is promising. In practice, the location of the tear, its size, the quality of the meniscus, and the stability of the repair affect the rehabilitation to be applied to the athlete. Neuromuscular control is very important in current rehabilitation. The individual needs and sports-specific approaches of the athlete should not be ignored in rehabilitation.

Meniscal tears in young athletes have great challenges for orthopedists. High activity-level, long career expectancy requires all conditions to be repaired. The high potential of recovery according to adults is an important advantage.

Athletes may be asked to be guided by the orthopedist athlete or club when planning treatment. Often, the athlete's desire to return to sports early can create pressure on the physician. The rehabilitation process following the treatment of accompanying ligamentous injuries gives the physician the time required for recovery after meniscus repair. However, the expectation of early sports return to isolated meniscus tears may force the physician to perform meniscectomy. Taking into account the expectations of the athlete and the situation in which he/she is not affected from the orthopedic pressures, it is to make the right decision to give priority to anatomical and functional meniscus repair.

Meniscal Rasping

Meniscal rasping is used to clean the torn edges of the meniscus to stimulate bleeding. It is indicated in patients with stable, longitudinal tears in the vascular region of the meniscus. In the case of unstable knee or avascular region ruptures, this treatment is not appropriate.

Meniscal Suturing

Red-red zone or red-white zone tears can be repaired. Traditionally, longitudinal tears are most suitable for suturing and healing. The most important condition for a good recovery is a stable knee. Repair of meniscus in unstable knees results in failure of treatment.

However, a stable knee with normal kinematics does not apply unnecessary shear force on the meniscus repair. Recently, positive results have been obtained regarding the repair of full-thickness radial tears. The results of the repair were not reported in randomized controlled trials. However, case reports seem to be positive. Repairs in the avascular region are at risk of failure. Meniscus repair, with ACL reconstruction, showed better recovery rates than ACL stable knees.

Meniscal Suturing Techniques

Various techniques for the repair of meniscus have been described:

Outside-in Meniscal Suturing Techniques

It was the first arthroscopic node technique. It is now the least used method. Suitable for tears in the middle and anterior 1/3 section of the meniscus. Posterior 1/3 cut is not possible with this technique.

The most important advantages of the outside-in repair method are that it is very easy to reach the anterior 1/3 region ruptures which are difficult to reach by other methods and it does not require additional posteromedial or posterolateral cuts to protect the vascular nerve pack. The most important disadvantage of this method is the difficulty in reaching tears extending to the posterior 1/3.

Inside-out Meniscal Suturing Techniques

Single- or double-lumen, special-inclined cannula through the needles passed through the repair. It can be applied to tears in every region, but it is more suitable for tears in the rear and middle 1/3 section. With this method, which is accepted as the gold standard in meniscus repair, the desired number and type of stitches can be placed easily in each region of the meniscus.

The most important disadvantage of the method is the need for a second incision in the posteromedial or posterolateral to prevent the needles from the capsule from causing vascular nerve injury, requiring an experienced assistant and special instrumentation.

The repair of tears near the posterior insertion of the meniscus is difficult and dangerous with the inside-out technique. In this type of tear, Morgan described the whole technique of sewing inside.

Meniscus Fixators

Implants called "meniscus fixators" have been developed due to the difficulties of sewing techniques, in some cases requiring additional incisions and vascular nerve complications. These implants manufactured as arrow, hook, anchor, screw, or staple are biodegradable or permanent.

The most important advantage of the fixators is that they are technically very easy. In addition, there are advantages such as very low vascular nerve complications, no need for additional incisions, meniscus tears in hard-to-reach areas, "all-in-one" repair, no assistant, and no need for arthroscopic nodes. Generally, there is no problem in the visualization of the lateral compartment. Medial repair on very narrow knees can be difficult.

However, the fixators have serious disadvantages. The mechanical forces are half or one-third of the vertical stitch.

Another problem with meniscus fixators is the risk of rigid implants to damage the articular cartilage. This problem arises especially in puffy head implants, which are not fully embedded in the meniscus body.

Methods for improving healing in tears extending to the nonvascular area have been described:

- Fibrin clot technique: When the patient's venous blood is mixed with a glass baguette, the paste-shaped clot is placed between the torn lips. Since Arnoczky showed the chemotactic and mitogenic factors involved in these dogs and showed that this clot had a positive effect on healing, this technique was also introduced in humans.
- Trephination technique: This method is based on the principle of opening radial tunnels in the meniscus body so that the peripheral vascular structures reach the avascular region. Zhang et al. showed that the trephination combined with the suture was more effective than the suture alone in avascular tears in the goat meniscus.

Synovial Abrasion

It is based on the principle of a hemorrhage and infusion responses as a result of filing the synovial tissue around the rupture with the help of a curette and contributing to the healing process.

Synovial Flap Transfer

It was shown that a better repair tissue was formed in the animal experiments with the interposition of a vascular tissue, a pedicled flap, in the tear area of the synovium. However, this technique has not been widely used.

Texture Adhesives

An ideal tissue adhesive should include the following: Tissue compatibility, biodegradable, good connect, minimal tissue reaction, and affordable.

Tissue adhesives currently used in clinical practice are limited because they contain all of these features.

Growth Factors in Meniscus Repair

It is known that fibrin clots placed in meniscus tears increase the healing potential of these lesions. It has been shown that meniscal fibrochondrocytes have the ability to make matrix and cell proliferation when they are associated with mitogenic and chemotactic factors in wound hematoma. In fibrochondrocyte cell culture, platelet-derived growth factor (PDGF) has been shown to stimulate proliferation of these cells.

Researchers showed that PDGF alone could not initiate meniscus repair in the central region of the meniscus.

The effect of endothelial cell growth factor (ECGF) on the healing potential of meniscal injuries was investigated. It has been said that there is not much effect.

Rehabilitation in Patients with Meniscus Repair

There is no consensus on knee movement, weight-bearing, knee pad use, and return to sports. In more conservative protocols, there are 4–6 weeks of partial load, knee movements gradually increased in knee pad control, and 6 months of deep crouching and sports ban. In contrast, aggressive protocols recommend immediate burdening, unlimited knee movement, and return to sports when muscle strength is acquired, as long as the patient can tolerate it.

In 95 patients with aggressive and conservative protocols, there was no difference in failure rates. Since the only factor affecting the success of the repair is not rehabilitation, the results of various series are difficult to compare. The generally accepted opinion is that rehabilitation using only meniscus fixators is a little more conservative.

Scaffolds

Scaffolds can be used as salvage interventions in meniscus ruptures with irreparable meniscus tears and athletes with segmental meniscectomy. The porous and absorbable structure should provide a meniscus-like tissue formation, while the biomechanical strength of the joint should be adequate.

In a European-centered study, 52 partial meniscectomy patients underwent polyurethane scaffold. In the third month, 81.4% of the patients underwent MRI. In the 12th month of the arthroscopic evaluation, in 97.7% of the cases, scaffold integration was detected with real meniscus tissue. Zaffagnini et al. 43 patients with lateral menisectomy applied scaffold. At the sixth postoperative month, they showed functional improvement. At the 12th month, the knee swelling and fatigue decreased to the optimal level. At the 24-month follow-up, 58% of the cases had reached the pre-injury activity level, and 95% of the patients had patient satisfaction.

However, it is recommended not to give a full load for 6–8 weeks after meniscus scaffold applications. This causes muscle atrophy especially in athletes and is inadequate to prevent rehabilitation muscle atrophy.

Nowadays, cell scaffolds have been introduced. The benefit of cell-free scaffolds was questioned. The factors affecting the success of the procedure were indicated as chronicity of the injury, body mass index, and other accompanying knee problems. Long-term studies on the results of scaffold applications, especially in athletes, are needed.

Meniscus Transplantation

Meniscus transplantation has been proposed to prevent the development of arthrosis in young patients whose meniscus is completely removed, without axial impairment and arthritic changes. The structures used for meniscus replacement in experimental and clinical studies are as follows: autografts, allografts, xenografts, synthetic polymer implants, carbon fiber and polyurethane implants.

It is doubtful that structures used as meniscus transplant may prevent the development of arthritis in the knee in the long term.

Allograft Transplantation

Subtotal or total meniscectomy after the functional deficiency and pain is applied in athletes. After close meniscectomy, especially under the influence of abnormal load distribution in the lateral compartment, chondral lesions develop in the early period. The rehabilitation of an athlete who develops a chondral lesion is more difficult, and in the late period, arthrosis develops frequently. For success in transplantation, it is important that the articular cartilage surface is smooth, stable, and normal or that BMI is below 30. In a recent meta-analysis, good and excellent results were reported in 84% of cases after transplantation.

Again in a recent study, posttransplantation in 12 professional footballers was performed in 92% of the cases. At the 36th month, 75% of the cases were reported to continue their professional sports lives.

Studies and discussions on transplantation still continue, with short-term to midterm results being positive. There is a rare risk of infection. The delay in returning to sports due to the long healing process is the biggest obstacle to the technique. Currently, randomized controlled long-term studies are needed.

It should be kept in mind that this intervention can be applied after the professionalism of the athletes who have undergone meniscectomy in their careers and who are symptomatic or postponed transplantation in their careers.

Calf Strain

A calf strain is a tear to one or more of the muscles at the back of the lower leg.

Calf Strain Symptoms

Symptoms of a calf strain vary significantly depending on how bad your injury is:

- A mild strain may feel more like an ache during or after exercise.
- With a more severe strain, you will feel a sudden sharp pain at the back of the lower leg at the time of injury.
- Calf muscle strains are graded from 1 to 3, with grade 3 being the most severe.

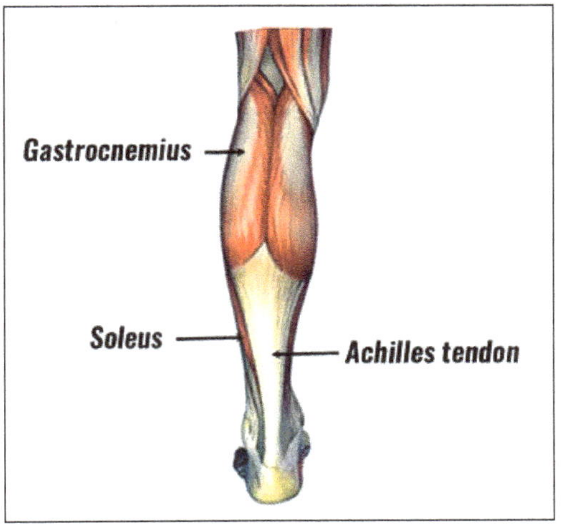

A Calf strain is simply a tear of one of the muscles which make up the calf muscle group at the back of the lower leg. The calf muscle group consists of the Gastrocnemius and Soleus muscles.The gastrocnemius is the big muscle at the back of the lower leg. The soleus is the smaller of the two and is located lower down and lies underneath the gastrocnemius.

Both muscles contract to produce 'plantar flexion' at the ankle joint. This is the same movement as standing up onto your tip-toes. The Gastrocnemius is the more powerful muscle which produces propulsion during dynamic movements such as sprinting and jumping.

Tennis Leg

The most common type of calf strain is a tear to the medial (inside) part of the gastrocnemius muscle. This is often referred to as 'Tennis leg' because it was so common in Tennis players. In particular, the musculotendinous junction (MTJ), where the tendon joins the muscle belly is a very common area to be injured.

Causes of Torn Calf Muscle

Calf muscle strains usually occur either as a result of a sudden, pushing off movement, or from excessive and forced over-stretching of the muscles. This is more likely to occur from a sudden explosive change of direction. However, there are factors which increase the chances of sustaining a torn calf muscle:

- Not warming up properly. If your muscles are particularly tight, then they may be more susceptible to injury.
- Athletes who have chronic shortening of the calf muscles, either from congenital reasons (genetics), or poor footwear choices.
- Wearing high heels regularly increases the risk of a number of injuries including calf muscle injuries. The muscles adaptively shorten over time and as a result, are strengthened in a contracted state. When the athlete wears flat running shoes they over-stretch, increasing the risk of a torn muscle.

Calf Strain Treatment

Treatment involves immediate first aid, followed by active rest, stretching and strengthening exercises.

Self-help Treatment

Immediate first aid is to apply the Apply the P.R.I.C.E. principles of protection rest, ice, compression and elevation as soon as possible.

- Protect your muscle from further damage. Stop playing or running.
- Rest: In the early acute stage complete rest is best. Once the acute phase has passed then active rest may be more benefitial than complete rest. However, stoppiong activities such as running and playing sport are advised at least until walking is pain-free. There is evidence to support the theory that muscles heal with some stress, but this must be controlled. If in any doubt, 'less is best'.
- Ice: Use a cold therapy and compression wrap to minimise any bleeding within the muscle. Cold therapy can be applied for 10 to 15 minutes every hour initially, reducing frequency as symptoms allow. Do not apply ice directly to the skin as it can cause ice burns.
- Compression: Wear a compression bandage or calf support to support the muscle and reduce swelling. Compressing blood vessels in the muscle encourages swelling to drain away from the area. In the later stages, when running and agility exercises are introduced, a heat retainer type support can be worn. This will help keep the muscle warm and improve blood flow.

- Heel lift: Wear a heel pad in your shoes. This shortens the muscle, reducing the load on it. Place in both shoes otherwise one leg will be longer than the other. Later, when you return to running, remove them to avoid adaptive muscle shortening.
- Exercises: When pain allows, begin gentle stretching and strengthening exercises.
- Foam roller: In the later stages of rehabilitation, a foam roller may be used to help mobilise the muscle and fascia.

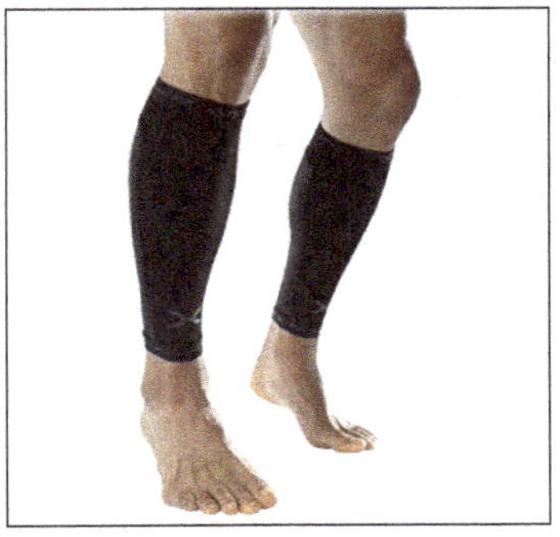

Exercises for Calf Strains

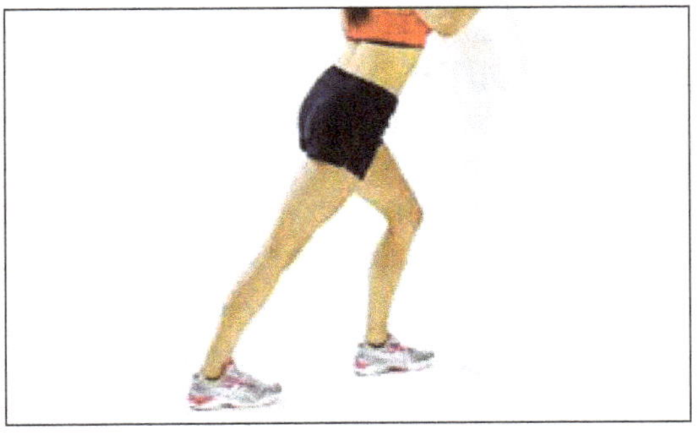

Both stretching and strengthening exercises are important for calf injuries. Exercises should only begin after the acute stage of healing has passed and always be performed pain-free.

- Active calf stretches are recommended once the early stages of recovery have been completed. They involve moving your foot yourself to stretch the muscles.
- As your muscle heals, static stretches should be done with the leg both straight and bent to target both the gastrocnemius and soleus muscles.
- Strengthening exercises can also begin as soon as pain allows. Plantar flexion with a resistance band is a gentle exercise, to begin with, along with seated calf raises.

- Eventually, more dynamic, functional exercises bridge the gap between basic rehab exercises and full fitness.

Rehabilitation of Ankle and Foot Injuries in Athletes

The foot and ankle are among the most common sites for both acute and chronic injuries in athletes and other physically active individuals. Although seldom life-threatening, they often have detrimental effects on sport activity and participation. When an injury to the foot or ankle occurs athletes are limited in their abilities to run, jump, kick, and change directions. Thus, the treatment and rehabilitation of these injuries are crucial in returning athletes to full participation at full functioning. When managing injuries for the foot and ankle, all of the typical clinical considerations must be thought of (type of injury, severity, healing time, type and level of activity, etc), but it is also important to consider other factors such as foot type, biomechanics, footwear worn during activity, and external supports such as bracing or taping. The foot is the base of the lower quarter kinetic chain, thus if rehabilitation and treatment is not managed properly, an injury to the foot or ankle can ultimately cause secondary injuries elsewhere up the chain.

Biomechanics of Normal Walking

For all sports medicine specialists, evaluation of gait is important for the rehabilitation of lower extremity injuries. Understanding the normal gait pattern will enable a clinician to identify and correct improper compensations after injury. The identification of gait abnormalities should play a key component in deciding to refer a patient for supervised rehabilitation. The movement of the lower extremity during normal walking and running can be divided into two phases, the stance phase and the swing phase.

The stance or support phase, starts with initial contact at heel strike and ends at toe-off. This phase has two important functions. First, at heel strike, the foot acts like a shock absorber to the impact forces and then the foot adapts to the surface. Secondly, at toe-off the foot functions as a rigid level to transmit the force from the foot to the surface. At initial contact, the subtalar joint is supinated and there is an external rotation of the tibia. As the foot loads, the subtalar joint moves into a pronated position until the forefoot is in contact with the ground. The change in subtalar motion occurs between initial heel strike and 20 percent into the support phase of running. As pronation occurs at the subtalar joint the tibia will rotate internally. Transverse plane rotation occurs at the knee joint because of this tibial rotation. Pronation of the foot unlocks the midtarsal joint and allows the foot to assist in shock absorption and to adapt to the uneven surfaces. It is important during initial impract to reduce the ground reaction forces and to distribute the load evenly on many different anatomical structures throughout the foot and leg. Pronation is normal and allows for this distribution of forces on as many structures as possible to avoid excessive loading on just a few structures. The subtalar joint remains in a pronated position until 55 to 85 percent of the support phase with maximam pronation is concurrent with the body's center of gravity passing over the base of support. From 70 to 90 percent of the support phase, the foot begins to resupinate and will approach the neutral subtalar position. In supination the midtarsal joints are locked and the foot becomes stable and rigid to prepare for push-off. This rigid position allows the foot to exert a greater amount of force from the lower extremity to the surface. The swing phase begins immediately after toe-off and ends as just prior to heel-strike. During the swing phase the leg is moved from behind the body to a position in front of the body.

Lateral Ankle Sprain

Lateral ankle sprains are common acute injuries suffered by athletes. The most common mechanism for a lateral ankle sprain is excessive inversion and plantar flexion of the reafoot on the tibia. The injured ligaments are located on the lateral aspect of the ankle and include the anterior talofibular, the posterior talofibular, and the calcaneofibular.

With lateral ankle sprains, the severity of the ligament damage will determine the classification and course of treatment. In a grade 1 sprain, there is stretching of the ligaments with little or no joint instability. Pain and swelling for a grade 1 sprain are often mild and seldom debilitating. After initial management for pain and swelling of the grade 1 sprain, rehabilitation can often be started immediately. Time loss from physical activity for a grade 1 sprain is typically less than one week. Grade 2 sprains occur with some tearing of ligamentous fibers and moderate instability of the joint. Pain and swelling are moderate to severe and often immobilization is required for several days. With a grade 3 sprain, there is total rupture of the ligament with gross instability of the joint. Pain and swelling is so debilitating that weight bearing is impossible for up to several weeks.

Rehabilitation Expectations

With lateral ankle sprains regaining full range of motion, strength, and neuromuscular coordination are paramount during rehabilitation. Isometrics and open-chain range of motion can be completed by those patients who are non-weight bearing. Range of motion should focus on dorsiflexion and plantar flexion and be performed passively and actively as tolerated. During early rehabilitation, towel stretches, and wobble board range of motion should be introduced as tolerated. Stationary biking can aid dorsiflexion and plantar flexion motion in a controlled environment while also providing a cardiovascular workout for the athlete. Clinicians can also incorporate joint mobilizations to aid in dorsiflexion range of motion. Hydrotherapy is an excellent means to work on range of motion while also gaining the benefits of hydrostatic pressure.

Once weight bearing is tolerated, middle stage rehabilitation is started. This includes balance and neuromuscular control exercises as well as continued range of motion exercises as tolerated. Balance activities should progress from double-limbed stance to single-limb stance as well as from a firm surface to progressively more unstable surfaces. Closing the eyes or incorporating perturbations can further challenge patients. Patients can be asked to throw and catch weighted balls, perform single leg squats, and perform single limb balance and reaching exercises. Regaining and maintaining range of motion should be continued. Wobble board training and slant board stretches are also important to focus on heel cord stretching.

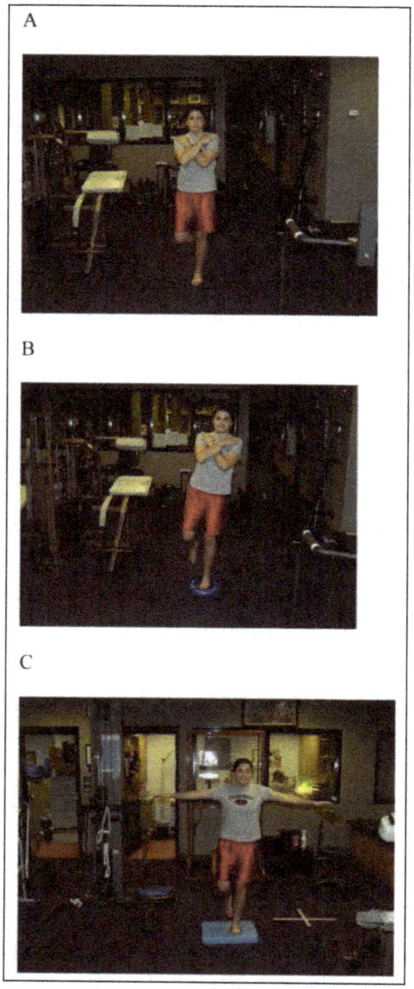

Balance training exercises include single limb standing. These exercises can be progressed by changing arm position, closing the eyes, and adding an unstable surface under the foot.

Increased strengthening exercises should be started once swelling and pain is controlled. Initially, dorsiflexion and plantar flexion strength should be focused on. Weight bearing calf raises and squats are examples excellent beginning exercises. As the ligaments heal, inversion and eversion strengthening should be added as tolerated.

Resistance bands and ankle weights are a good means to gain strength in all planes of motion. Clinicians can integrate diagonal exercises (ie, combined plantar flexion/inversion and dorsiflexion/eversion) to isolate motions at the talocrural joint.

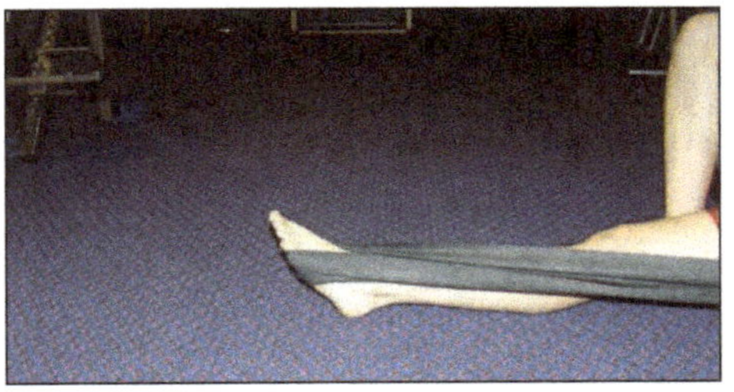

Strength training may be performed with resistance tubing exercises.

During this time, it is paramount for clinicians to re-educate athletes on the proper mechanics of walking. Once range of motion and strength is regained, functional activities are included. Functional rehabilitation exercises should begin with simple, uniplaner exercises; walking and jogging in a straight line. Once the athlete can perform these without a pain or a limp, hops, jumps, skips and change of direction can start to be added. Have the athlete perform 10 jumps for distance on the uninvolved limb and challenge him/her to match the distance with the involved limb. Do the same for jumps for height. As cutting is started, begin with wide arching turns and progress to tighter, sharper and faster cuts. Athletes should be challenged to perform lateral movements as well such as shuffling and carioca. As the patient becomes more comfortable and functional, have him/her perform rehab wearing the typical shoe/cleat for the sport and progress to more sport specific activities.

Depending on the severity of the ankle sprain, fear avoidance may cause the athlete to alter play and be at higher risk for reinjury or injury to another location. Also, some sport-specific skills may need to be reconditioned. Participation into sport should start with non-contact drills and progress to contact drills and finally to full scrimmage.

Criteria for Full Competition

Full return to activity should be a gradual progression in order to stress the ligaments without causing further harm. Full activity should be allowed once the athlete has complete range of motion, 80 to 90 percent of preinjury strength, and a normal gait pattern including the ability to perform sport-specific tasks such as cutting and landing without any compensations due to the injury. The athlete should be capable, without pain or swelling to complete a full practice.

Clinical Pearls

- Challenge patients with home-exercises: Have them try to balance on involved limb while brushing teeth, progress to eyes shut while brushing their teeth and balancing.

- Have rehabilitation clinicians perform talocrural and tibiofibular joint mobilizations to increase dorsiflexion.
- Perform exercises with shoes on and off to alter the planter cutaneous feedback.
- Using a 10-20 yard area, have the patient walk on toes back in forth. Repeat walking with toes pointed in, toes pointed out, and on heels (toes in the air).
- Ask the subject to perform 10 single leg jumps in a row on the involved limb as high as possible in a row, while watching his/her face, if he/she can complete without grimacing safe to start functional rehabilitation.

Patient Education

The leading predisposing factor for an ankle sprain is a history of an ankle sprain and an estimated 30% of all individuals who suffer an initial ankle sprain will develop chronic ankle instability. Thus, patients need to know that inadequate treatment and rehabilitation of an ankle sprain has a great likelihood of leading to future problems.

Often patients, coaches, and parents have the mindset that a lateral ankle sprain is not serious and players can return quickly. In fact, in many cases health care services are not even sought by individuals suffering an ankle sprain. It is critical for all stakeholders to understand the high frequency of residual symptoms and recurrent sprains. The importance of allowing the ligaments to heal, regaining full range of motion, strength, and balance prior to returning to activity must be emphasized to patients. If, while doing rehabilitation swelling returns, patients must know that they did too much.

Prophylactic Support

Prophylactic support is often used after an ankle sprain to provide mechanical stability. Depending upon individual preference and budget, athletes can use tape or a variety of braces (lace-up, stirrup, or elastic type of configuration. Both taping and bracing have been found to reduce the risk of recurrent ankle sprains in athletes. Advantages of a braces include easy of application and cost effectiveness. Braces also provide the athlete with proprioceptive stimulation, which implies an improve proprioception and sensory feedback. Taping, one the other hand can be custom designed for the specific athlete, sport, and instabilities.

Other Ankle Sprains

Although less common, medial and syndesmodic ankle sprains often result in more severe injuries causing longer time to heal and rehabilitate. Medial ankle sprains occur with a mechanism of excessive eversion and dorsiflexion, causing the deltoid ligament to be injured. Patients with medial ankle sprains will often present with swelling and discoloration on the medial aspect of the ankle and unwillingness to bear weight.

Syndesmodic sprains occur with disruption of the interosseous (or syndesmodic) ligament that stabilizing the inferior tibiofibular joint. Injury to this ligament occurs with excessive external rotational or forced dorsiflexion. Syndesmotic sprains may occur in isolation or in combination with medial or lateral ankle sprains. Due to limited blood supply and the difficulty in allowing the injured ligament to heal unless the ankle is immobilized, injuries to the syndesmodic ligaments often take months to heal. Patients with syndesmodic sprains often present with a lack of swelling, but will be extremely tender over anterior aspect of the distal tibiofibular joint.

Rehabilitation Expectations

Initial treatment for both medial and syndesmodic sprains is often immobilization and crutches. During this time, swelling and pain management are the primary concerns. The length of time of immobilization will vary among patients and will depend on the severity of the sprain. While immobilized, patients can work on controlled open-chain range of motion, focusing on dorsiflexion and plantar flexion. During this time, inversion and eversion should be held to a minimum. During early rehabilitation, nothing should increase pain or swelling to the area.

Once weight-bearing is tolerated, crutches should be used at a minimum. Gait training may be needed to ensure the patient is not compensating in any way, which may cause secondary injury. Rehabilitation concerns include; pain and swelling, range of motion, strength, balance and neuromuscular control, and functional exercises.

Criteria for Full Competition

Full return to activity should be a gradual progression in order to stress the ligaments without causing further harm. Full activity should be allowed once the athlete has complete range of motion, 80 to 90 percent of preinjury strength, and the ability to perform gait activities (including running and changing direction) without difficulty. The athlete should be capable, without pain or swelling to complete a full practice.

With medial and syndesmodic sprains, patience is the most important thing for the patient to learn. The healing of the medial and syndesmodic ligaments take time, sometimes up to severalmonths to fully heal. The difference in the expectations of these injuries compared to lateral ankle sprains must be emphasized to all stakeholders so that realistic expectations for return to play can be understood.

Plantar Fasciitis

Plantar fasciitis is the catchall term that is commonly used to describe pain on the plantar aspect of the proximal arch and heel. The plantar fascia is an aporneurosis that runs the length of the sole of the foot and is a broad dense band of connective tissue. It is attached proximally to the medial surface of the calcaneus and fans out distally, attaching to the metatarsophalangeal articulations and merges into the capsular ligaments.

The plantar aponeurosis assists in maintaining the stability of the foot and secures or braces the longitudinal arch.

Plantar fasciitis is caused by a straining of the fascia near its origin. The plantar fascia is under tension with toe extension and depression of the longitudinal arch. During normal standing (weight bearing principally on the heel), the fascia is under minimal stress, however, when the weight is shifted to the balls of the feet (running) the fascia is put under stress and strain. Often planar fasciitis is a result of chronic running with poor technique, poor footwear, or because of lordosis, a condition in which the increased forward tilt of the pelvis produces an unfavorable angle of foot-strike when there is considerable force exerted on the ball of the foot.

Patients more prone to plantar fasciitis include: those with a pes cavus foot; excessive pronation; overweight; walking , running or standing for long periods of time, especially on hard surfaces; old, worn shoes (insufficient arch support); and tight Achilles tendon. The patient will present with pain in the anterior medial heel, usually at the attachment of the plantar fascia to the calcaneus. The pain is particularly noticeable during the first couple of steps in the morning or after sitting for a long time. Often the pain will lessen as the patient moves more, however the pain will increase if the athlete is on his/her feet excessively or on his/her toes often. Upon inspection, the plantar fascia may or may not be swollen with crepitus. The patient's pain will increase with forefoot and toe dorsiflexion.

Rehabilitation Expectations

Depending on patient compliance, plantar fasciitis can be a very treatable minor injury with symptoms lasting days. However, without proper treatment and patient compliance, plantar fasciitis can linger for months or even years.

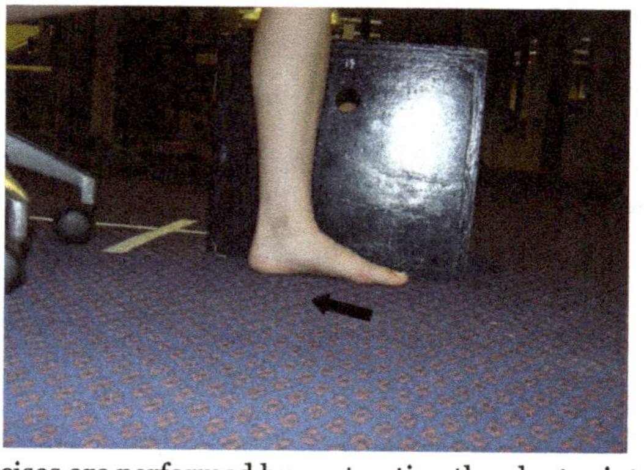

Short foot exercises are performed by contracting the plantar intrinsic muscles in an effort to pull the metatarsal heads towards the calcaneus. Emphasis should be placed on minimizing extrinsic muscle activity.

Initial treatment of plantar fasciitis starts with pain control. Rest is extremely important at this time, patients should not being performing any unnecessary weight bearing.

Patients should also be wearing comfortable supportive shoes when walking is necessary. Adding a heel cup or custom foot orthosis to a patient's shoe may relieve some of the pain at the plantar fascia insertion. During this time, regaining full dorsiflexion range of motion of the foot as well as of the big toe is vital. Towel stretches, slant board stretches, and joint mobilizations administered by a rehabilitation clinician will aid in the return of dorsiflexion range of motion.

After pain is reduced strengthening exercises can be incorporated into rehabilitatoin. The focus should be in strengthening some of the smaller extrinsic and intrinsic muscles of the foot. Towel crutches, big toe-little toes raises, short foot exercises are good examples of strengthening exercises. Throughout the treatment and rehabilitation process, soft tissue work such as cross-friction massage may aid in the alleviation of symptoms.

Criteria for Full Competition

Although athletes can often continue to participate fully while suffering from plantar fasciitis, it should be understood that the longer activity is continued, the longer the symptoms will linger. For best recovery of this injury, extra activity should not be started until the athlete is able to walk a full day without any pain. Once a daily activities are tolerated, activity can slowly be increased until full participation. Throughout the rehabilitation and participation progression stretching should occur often throughout the day.

Clinical Pearls

- While sitting, roll on a ball (tennis ball, golf ball, etc) underneath the medial longitudinal to stretch the plantar fascia.
- Fill a paper cup with water and freeze it, roll on the frozen cup to get the benefits of cold while also stretching the plantar fascia.
- Before getting out of bed in the morning, but on shoes with good arch supports to provide the plantar fascia support upon weight-bearing.
- Sleep with feet off the end of the bed to allow some dorsiflexion while sleeping.
- Wear a night splint that will keep foot in a dorsiflexed or neutral position.
- Stretching often throughout the day for a short period of time is more beneficial then stretching once a day for a long period of time.
- Do not weight high-heels or other shoes with no support (sandals) during the day.

Patient Education

Plantar fascia tends to be a cyclical injury. Athletes will repetitively suffer from this injury because after the initial injury, the cause of the injury is not treated, only the symptoms. Patients with plantar fasciitis need to have their gait biomechanics thoroughly evaluated and, if necessary, be fitted for custom orthotics.

Achilles Tendonitis

Achilles tendonitis is an inflammatory condition that involves the Achilles tendon and/or its tendon sheath. Achilles tendonitis is the most common overuse injuries reported in distance runners. Although Achilles tendonitis is generally a chronic condition, acute injury may also occur. Typically, the athlete will suffer from gradual pain and stiffness about the Achilles tendon region, 2 to 6 cm proximal to the calcaneal insertion. The pain will increase after running hills, stairs, or an increased amount of sprints (running on toes). Upon evaluation, the gastrocnemius and soleus muscle testing may be normal however, flexibility will be reduced. Having the patient perform toe raises to fatigue will show a deficit compared to the uninvolved limb. Inspection of the area may feel warm to the touch and pain, tenderness and crepitus may be felt with palpation. The tendon may appear thickened indicating a chronic condition.

Rehabilitation Expectations

Healing of Achilles tendonitis is a slow process due to the lack of vascularity to the tendon. Initially, patients will feel comfortable by placing less stress to the area by wearing a heel cup. Resting and activity modification is important during the initially healing stages. The clinician needs to emphasize the importance of allowing the tendon to heal. During this time, cross friction massage can be started to the area to break down adhesions and promote blood flow to the area.

Stretching and strengthening of the gastrocnemious-soleus complex should be incorporated as tolerated by the patient. Towel stretching and slant board stretching should be done throughout the day. As range of motion is restored, the heel cup should be removed to reduce the chances of adaptive shortening of the muscles and tendon. Progressive strengthening including toe raises and resistive tubing should be incorporated at the beginning of rehabilitation. Sets should start low with low reps and gradually increase to low sets high reps for endurance as tolerated by the athlete. As pain and inflammation decreases, machine weights, lunges, and sport specific exercises can be added. Eccentric exercises for the triceps surae often have beneficial results in athletes with Achilles tendonitis.

The patient's foot structure and gait mechanics should be evaluated for possible orthotic benefits. Often Achilles tendonitis is a result of overpronation, an abnormality that can be addressed with foot orthoses. Once range of motion, strength and endurance has returned, athletes should slowly progress into walking and jogging program. Workouts should be done on a flat surface when possible. The walking and jogging program should start out with slow mini-bursts of speed. The program is to increase the amount of stress the Achilles tendon can tolerate; it is not to improve overall endurance. As tolerated by the patient, running and sprinting can be increased.

Criteria for Full Competition

Athletes should be allowed to compete when full range of motion and strength has returned. The athlete should have regained endurance in the involved limb and be capable of completing a full practice without pain. Depending on the sport, some athletes may be able to compete while suffering from Achilles tendonitis. However, patients should be educated in the fact that the condition will not go away without proper rest and treatment.

Patient Education

Patients need to be educated with the risks of Achilles tendonitis, specifically hill running, lack of proper shoes, lack of rest, and flexibility. Hill workouts increase the stress and strain to the gastrocnemius-soleus complex and Achilles tendon. Hill workouts should be done at a maximum once a week to allow the body time to heal. Similar to any chronic injury to the feet, shoes must be evaluated. Athletes need to learn and understand their foot type and the proper shoes for their foot type. Also, shoes should be replaced every 500 miles are a maximum 2 years. Running on old worn shoes will alter biomechanics and cause stress and strain to the body. Finally, the lack of flexibility is often the main culprit in Achilles tendonitis. The importance of stretching and stretching often should be emphasized.

Prophylactic Support

Initially, heel cups will reduce the tension and stress placed on the Achilles tendon. As flexibility is regained, the heel cup should be gradually reduced to reduce the chances of an adaptive shortening of the tendon. Athletes may find comfort in a special tape job that will reduce the stress placed on the Achilles tendon as well. The patient's foot type and gait mechanics should be evaluated for possible use of custom orthotics. Achilles tendonitis can often be attributed to over pronation during gait. A custom orthotic will be able to adjust the athlete's gait to reduce this abnormality.

Turf Toe

Tuft toe is a hyperextension injury of the great toe, causing a sprain to the metatarsophalangeal joint and damage to the joint capsule. Turf toe can be either an acute or a chronic condition. An acute turf toe often occurs when the athlete's shoe sticks into the ground while he/she is trying to stop quickly. The shoe sticks as the individual's body weight shifts forward, causing the big toe to jam into the shoe and ground. The chronic condition occurs from frequent running or jumping in shoes that allow excessive great toe motion. This mechanism of injury may occur on natural or synthetic surfaces.

Athletes with turf toe will present with pain at the 1st metatarsophalangeal joint. Swelling and stiffness may be present, however pain, especially with great toe extension is the primary symptom. Rehabilitation of turf toe typically requires several weeks. If left untreated, turf toe can lead to permanent decrease in range of motion and osteoarthritis arthritis.

Rehabilitation Concerns

Patients suffering from turf toe respond best with rest and an adjustment made to their shoes. Pain management should be of primary concern to the clinician. Once pain and swelling have been reduced, the athlete should start performing toe extension and flexion exercises such as toe crunches and short foot exercises. Joint mobilizations should be added to the treatment protocol to aid in pain and increase range of motion. Once pain and swelling is reduced, the athlete may begin to progress into athletic activities. Protecting the great toe with a stiff forefoot insert or a great toe taping may increase athlete comfort.

Criteria for Full Competition

Athletes are able to return to full competition when any pain and swelling has resolved. Often athletes with turf toe are capable to continue practicing and participating while suffering from this injury with the toe being taped and possible inserts into shoes.

Pearls of Wisdom

- Have patients wear stiff insoled shoes to prevent excessive motion.
- Great toe joint mobilizations can be incorporated to reduce pain and increase motion.

Patient Education

Patients should be aware that if left untreated, turf toe may cause permanent decreased range of motion in the great toe and bone spurs may develop. Although athletes can often play with turf toe, rest and pain management is the most beneficial for athletes. Without prevention of excessive extension of the great toe, symptoms of turf toe may disappear with rest just to return once the athlete returns to activity.

Prophylactic Support

Athletes with turf toe may benefit from adding a steel or other stiff material insert into the forefoot of the shoes to reduce extension. Taping of the great toe to prevent dorsiflexion may also be done.

References

- Shin-splints: physio-pedia.com, Retrieved 7 May, 2020
- Achilles-Tendon-Rehab-final-143151: uwhealth.org, Retrieved 21 July, 2020

- Combined-Patellar-Tendinitis: sportmed.com, Retrieved 15 January, 2020
- Hubbard, MJ; Hildebrand, BA; Battafarano, MM; Battafarano, DF (June 2018). "Common Soft Tissue Musculoskeletal Pain Disorders". Primary Care. 45 (2): 289–303. doi:10.1016/j.pop.2018.02.006. PMID 29759125
- Rotator-cuff-tendinitis, health: healthline.com, Retrieved 21 July, 2020
- Review-of-current-concepts-2329-9096.1000142: omicsonline.org, Retrieved 21 April, 2020
- Minassian, K; Hofstoetter, US; Danner, SM; Mayr, W; Bruce, JA; McKay, WB; Tansey, KE (March 2016). "Spinal Rhythm Generation by Step-Induced Feedback and Transcutaneous Posterior Root Stimulation in Complete Spinal Cord-Injured Individuals". Neurorehabilitation and Neural Repair. 30 (3): 233–43. doi:10.1177/1545968315591706. PMID 26089308
- Lower-back-pain, sports-medicine-conditions: upmc.com, Retrieved 17 April, 2020

Physical Therapies

4

- Manual Therapy
- Cryotherapy
- Dry Needling
- Chiropractic
- Aquatic Therapy
- Hydrotherapy
- Telerehabilitation
- Medicine Ball
- Diathermy
- Electrotherapy
- Gait Training
- Heat Therapy
- Splint
- Traction
- Soft Tissue Therapy

Physical therapies treat the deformities and some injuries by using different physical methods and specially designed exercises. It includes cryotherapy, dry needling, hydrotherapy, diathermy, electrotherapy, heat therapy, soft tissue therapy, etc. This chapter sheds light on the various physical therapies for a thorough understanding of the subject.

Manual Therapy

Manual therapy has a long history within the profession of physical therapy and physical therapists have greatly contributed to the current diversity in manual therapy approaches and techniques. Mechanical explanations were historically used to explain the mechanisms by which manual therapy interventions worked, new research reveals intricate neurophysiologic mechanisms are also at play and the beneficial psychological effects of providing hands-on examination and intervention should not be ignored.

The International Federation of Orthopaedic Manipulative Physical Therapists (IFOMPT) defines manual therapy techniques as: "Skilled hand movements intended to produce any or all of the following effects: improve tissue extensibility; increase range of motion of the joint complex; mobilize or manipulate soft tissues and joints; induce relaxation; change muscle function; modulate pain; and reduce soft tissue swelling, inflammation or movement restriction."

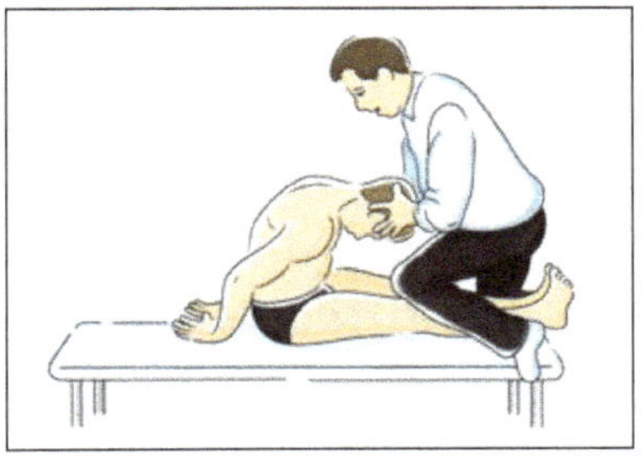

According the the American Academy of Orthopaedic Manual Physical Therapists (AAOMPT) Description of Advanced Specialty Practice (DASP), orthopaedic manual physical therapy (OMPT) is defined as: any "hands-on" treatment provided by the physical therapist.

Treatment may include moving joints in specific directions and at different speeds to regain movement (joint mobilization and manipulation), muscle stretching, passive movements of the affected body part, or having the patient move the body part against the therapist's resistance to improve muscle activation and timing. Selected specific soft tissue techniques may also be used to improve the mobility and function of tissue and muscles."

Three paradigms for manual therapy therapeutic effects:

- Physiological: Positive placebo response.
- Biomechanical and Physical: Facilitates repair and tissue modeling.
- Psychological: Pain relief via- stimulates gating mechanism; muscle inhibition; reduction of nocioceptive activity; reduced intraarticular or periarticular pressure.

Techniques Include

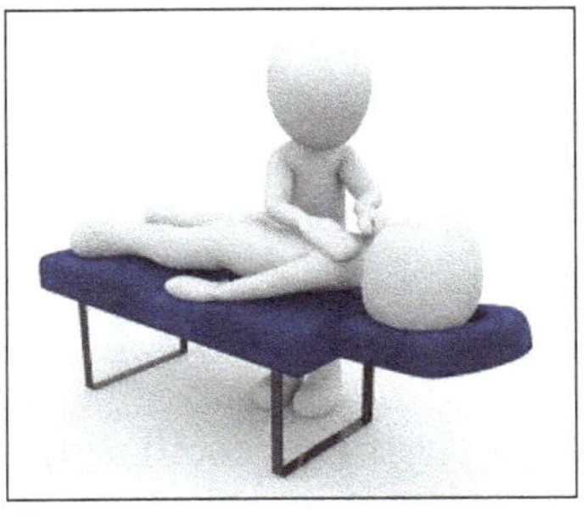

- Traction.
- Massage.

- Trigger Point Therapy.
- Active Release Techniques.
- Assisted Active Range of Motion (AAROM).
- Passive Range of Motion.
- Lymph Drainage.
- Stretches (muscle, neural tissue, joints, fascia).
- Instrument Assisted Soft Tissue Mobilization.
- Joint Manipulation: A passive, high velocity, low amplitude thrust applied to a joint complex within its anatomical limit* with the intent to restore optimal motion, function, and to reduce pain.
- Joint Mobilisation: A manual therapy technique comprising a continuum of skilled passive movements to the joint complex that are applied at varying speeds and amplitudes, that may include a small-amplitude/ high velocity therapeutic movement (manipulation) with the intent to restore optimal motion, function, and to reduce pain.

The terms "Thrust Manipulation" and "Non-Thrust Manipulation" have been used in the literature. "Thrust Manipulation" is used to describe interventions described as Manipulation by IFOMPT, and "Non-Thrust Manipulation" would be synonymous with the term Mobilization as proposed by IFOMPT.

Guide to Grading of Mobilisations/Manipulations

Maitland Joint Mobilization Grading Scale:

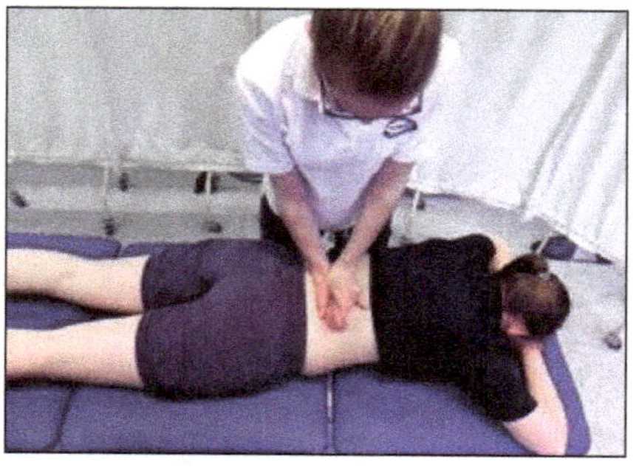

- Grade I - Small amplitude rhythmic oscillating mobilization in early range of movement.
- Grade II - Large amplitude rhythmic oscillating mobilization in midrange of movement.

- Grade III - Large amplitude rhythmic oscillating mobilization to point of limitation in range of movement.
- Grade IV - Small amplitude rhythmic oscillating mobilization at end of available range of movement.
- Grade V (Thrust Manipulation) - Small amplitude, quick thrust at end of available range of movement.

Kaltenborn Traction Grading Scale:

- Grade I - Neutralises joint pressure without separation of joint surfaces.
- Grade II - Separates articulating surfaces, taking up slack or eliminating play within joint capsule.
- Grade III - Stretching of soft tissue surrounding joint.

Joint Manipulation

Joint manipulation is a type of passive movement of a skeletal joint. It is usually aimed at one or more 'target' synovial joints with the aim of achieving a therapeutic effect.

Biomechanics

Manipulation can be distinguished from other manual therapy interventions such as joint mobilization by its biomechanics, both kinetics and kinematics.

Kinetics

Until recently, force-time histories measured during spinal manipulation were described as consisting of three distinct phases: the preload (or prethrust) phase, the thrust phase, and the resolution phase. Evans and Breen added a fourth 'orientation' phase to describe the period during which the patient is oriented into the appropriate position in preparation for the prethrust phase.

When individual peripheral synovial joints are manipulated, the distinct force-time phases that occur during spinal manipulation are not as evident. In particular, the rapid rate of change of force that occurs during the thrust phase when spinal joints are manipulated is not always necessary. Most studies to have measured forces used to manipulate peripheral joints, such as the metacarpophalangeal (MCP) joints, show no more than gradually increasing load. This is probably because there are many more tissues restraining a spinal motion segment than an independent MCP joint.

Kinematics

The kinematics of a complete spinal motion segment when one of its constituent spinal joints are manipulated are much more complex than the kinematics that occur during manipulation of an independent peripheral synovial joint. Even so, the motion that occurs between the articular surfaces of any individual synovial joint during manipulation should be very similar

Early models describing the kinematics of an individual target joint during the various phases of manipulation were based on studies that investigated joint cracking in MCP joints. The cracking was elicited by pulling the proximal phalanx away from the metacarpal bone (to separate, or 'gap' the articular surfaces of the MCP joint) with gradually increasing force until a sharp resistance, caused by the cohesive properties of synovial fluid, was met and then broken. These studies were therefore never designed to form models of therapeutic manipulation, and the models formed were erroneous in that they described the target joint as being configured at the end range of a rotation movement, during the orientation phase. The model then predicted that this end range position was maintained during the prethrust phase until the thrust phase where it was moved beyond the 'physiologic barrier' created by synovial fluid resistance; conveniently within the limits of anatomical integrity provided by restraining tissues such as the joint capsule and ligaments. This model still dominates the literature. However, after re-examining the original studies on which the kinematic models of joint manipulation were based, Evans and Breen argued that the optimal prethrust position is actually the equivalent of the neutral zone of the individual joint, which is the motion region of the joint where the passive osteoligamentous stability mechanisms exert little or no influence. This new model predicted that the physiologic barrier is only confronted when the articular surfaces of the joint are separated (gapped, rather than the rolling or sliding that usually occurs during physiological motion), and that it is more mechanically efficient to do this when the joint is near to its neutral configuration.

Cracking Joints

Joint manipulation is characteristically associated with the production of an audible 'clicking' or 'popping' sound. This sound is believed to be the result of a phenomenon known as cavitation occurring within the synovial fluid of the joint. When a manipulation is performed, the applied force separates the articular surfaces of a fully encapsulated synovial joint. This deforms the joint capsule and intra-articular tissues, which in turn creates a reduction in pressure within the joint cavity. In this low pressure environment, some of the gases that are dissolved in the synovial fluid (which are naturally found in all bodily fluids) leave solution creating a bubble or cavity, which rapidly collapses upon itself, resulting in a 'clicking' sound. The contents of this gas bubble are thought to be mainly carbon dioxide. The effects of this process will remain for a period of time termed the 'refractory period', which can range from a few minutes to more than an hour, while it is slowly reabsorbed back into the synovial fluid. There is some evidence that ligament laxity around the target joint is associated with an increased probability of cavitation.

Clinical Effects and Mechanisms of Action

The clinical effects of joint manipulation have been shown to include:

- Temporary relief of musculoskeletal pain.
- Shortened time to recover from acute back sprains (Rand).
- Temporary increase in passive range of motion (ROM).
- Physiological effects upon the central nervous system.
- No alteration of the position of the sacroiliac joint.

Common side effects of spinal manipulative therapy (SMT) are characterized as mild to moderate and may include: local discomfort, headache, tiredness, or radiating discomfort.

Shekelle summarised the published theories for mechanisms of action for how joint manipulation may exert its clinical effects as the following:

- Release of entrapped synovial folds or plica.
- Relaxation of hypertonic muscle.
- Disruption of articular or periarticular adhesions.
- Unbuckling of motion segments that have undergone disproportionate displacement.

Joint Mobilization

Joint mobilization is a manual therapy intervention, a type of straight-lined, passive movement of a skeletal joint that addresses arthrokinematic joint motion (joint gliding) rather than osteokinematic joint motion. It is usually aimed at a 'target' synovial joint with the aim of achieving a therapeutic effect. These techniques are used by a variety of health care professionals with specific training in manual therapy assessment and treatment techniques.

IFOMPT defines joint mobilization as "a manual therapy technique comprising a continuum of skilled passive movements that are applied at varying speeds and amplitudes to joints, muscles or nerves with the intent to restore optimal motion, function, and/or to reduce pain."

The APTA Guide to Physical Therapist Practice defines mobilization/manipulation as "a manual therapy technique comprised of a continuum of skilled passive movements that are applied at varying speeds and amplitudes, including a small amplitude/ high velocity therapeutic movement."

Classification and Mechanisms

Joint mobilization is classified by the Australian physiotherapist Geoffrey Douglas Maitland into five 'grades' of motion, each of which describes the range of motion of the target joint during the procedure. They are generally divided into five grades. The different grades of manipulation are known to produce selective activation of different mechanoreceptors in the joint.

- Grade I - Low amplitude, rhythmically oscillating joint glide near the resting position of the available arthrokinematic joint play. Activates Type I mechanoreceptors that inhibit nociception and provide information regarding joint position. They have a low threshold and respond to a few grams of tension.

Activates mechanoreceptors in the superficial layer of the joint capsule - Bulbous corpuscles.

- Grade II - Relatively large amplitude, rhythmically oscillating joint glide that carries well into the available arthrokinematic joint play. Activates Type II mechanoreceptors that inhibit nociception and provide information about joint acceleration. They also have a low threshold and respond to a few grams of tension.
- Activates mechanoreceptors in the deep layer of the joint capsule - Pacinian Corpuscles.
- Grade III - Relatively large amplitude, rhythmically oscillating joint glide that carries to the end of the available arthrokinematic joint play.
- Designed to physically stretch the joint capsule.
- Grade IV - Low amplitude, rhythmically oscillating joint glide that is performed at the end of the available arthrokinematic joint play.
- Designed to physically stretch the joint capsule.
- Grade V - This grade refers to the use of a single high-velocity, low-amplitude thrust performed at the end of the available joint play.

Activates Golgi tendon organ-like endings that inhibit muscle tone and monitor the direction of joint motion. They have a higher threshold and respond to forces on the order of kilograms - Golgi tendon organs.

Cryotherapy

Cryotherapy, sometimes known as cold therapy, is the local or general use of low temperatures in medical therapy. Cryotherapy may be used to treat a variety of tissue lesions. The most prominent use of the term refers to the surgical treatment, specifically known as cryosurgery or cryoablation. Cryosurgery is the application of extremely low temperatures to destroy abnormal or diseased tissue and is used most commonly to treat skin conditions.

Cryotherapy is used in an effort to relieve muscle pain, sprains and swelling after soft tissue damage or surgery. It can be a range of treatments from the application of ice packs or immersion in ice baths (generally known as cold therapy), to the use of cold chambers.

While cryotherapy is widely used, there is little evidence as to its efficacy that has been replicated or shown in large controlled studies. Its long term side effects have also not been studied.

Cryosurgery

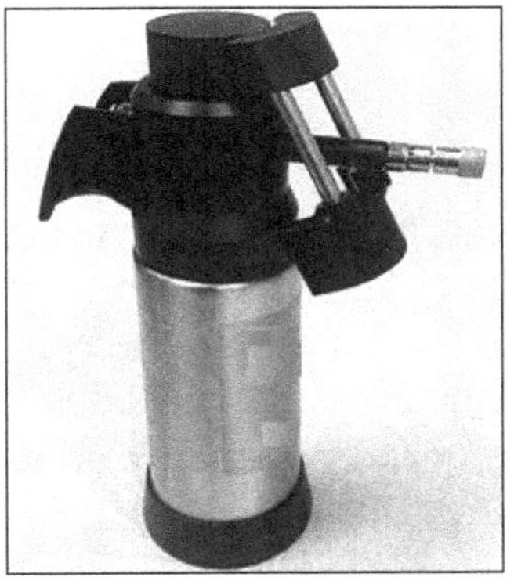

Medical cryotherapy gun.

Cryosurgery is the application of extreme cold to destroy abnormal or diseased tissue. The application of ultra-cold liquid causes damage to the treated tissue due to intracellular ice formation. The degree of damage depends upon the minimum temperature achieved and the rate of cooling. Cryosurgery is used to treat a number of diseases and disorders, most especially skin conditions like warts, moles, skin tags and solar keratoses. Liquid nitrogen is usually used to freeze the tissues at the cellular level. The procedure is used often as it is relatively easy and quick, can be done in the doctors surgery, and is deemed quite low risk. If a cancerous lesion is suspected then excision rather than cryosurgery may be deemed more appropriate.

Ice Pack Therapy

Ice pack therapy is a treatment of cold temperatures to an injured area of the body. Though the therapy is extensively used, and it is agreed that it alleviates symptoms, testing has produced conflicting results about its efficacy.

An ice pack is placed over an injured area and is intended to absorb heat of a closed traumatic or edematous injury by using conduction to transfer thermal energy. The physiologic effects of cold application include immediate vasoconstriction with reflexive vasodilation, decreased local metabolism and enzymatic activity, and decreased oxygen demand. Cold decreases muscle spindle fiber activity and slows nerve conduction velocity, therefore it is often used to decrease spasticity and muscle guarding. It is commonly used to alleviate the pain of minor injuries, as well as decrease muscle soreness. The use of ice packs in treatment decreases the blood flow most rapidly at the beginning of the cooling period, this occurs as a result of vasoconstriction, the initial reflex sympathetic activity.

Ice is not commonly used prior to rehabilitation or performance because of its known adverse effects to performance such as decreased myotatic reflex and force production, as well as a decrease in balance immediately following ice pack therapy for 20 minutes. However, if ice pack therapy is applied for less than 10 minutes, performance can occur without detrimental effects. If the ice pack is removed at this time, athletes are sent back to training or competition directly with no decrease in performance.

Cold Spray Anesthetics

In addition to their use in cryosurgery, several types of cold aerosol sprays are used for short-term pain relief. Ordinary spray cans containing tetrafluoroethane, dimethyl ether, or similar substances, are used to numb the skin prior to or possibly in place of local anesthetic injections, and prior to other needles, small incisions, sutures, and so on. Other products containing chloroethane are used to ease sports injuries, similar to ice pack therapy.

Whole Body Cryotherapy

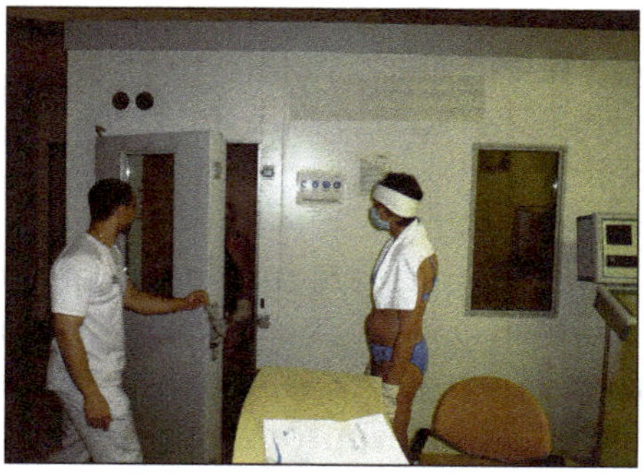

Cryotherapy patients during preparation of treatment of c. 3 minutes.

It is unclear if whole body cryotherapy (WBC) has any effect on muscle soreness, or improves recovery, after exercise. There is no evidence that whole body cooling effectively treats Alzheimer's, fibromyalgia, migraines, rheumatoid arthritis, multiple sclerosis, stress, anxiety, or chronic pain as its proponents claim.

This treatment involves exposing individuals to extremely cold dry air (below −100 °C) for two to four minutes. To achieve the subzero temperatures required for WBC, two methods are typically used: liquid nitrogen and refrigerated cold air. During these exposures, individuals wear minimal clothing, which usually consists of shorts for males, and shorts and a crop top for females. Gloves, a woollen headband covering the ears, and a nose and mouth mask, in addition to dry shoes and socks, are commonly worn to reduce the risk of cold-related injury. The first WBC chamber was built in Japan in the late 1970s, introduced to Europe in the 1980s, and has been used in the US and Australia in the past decade.

Adverse Effects

Reviews of whole body cryotherapy have called for research studies to implement active surveillance of adverse events, which are suspected of being underreported. If the cold temperatures are produced by evaporating liquid nitrogen, there is the risk of inert gas asphyxiation as well as frostbite.

Partial Body

Partial body cryotherapy (PBC) devices also exist. If the cold temperatures are produced by evaporating liquid nitrogen, there is the risk of inert gas asphyxiation as well as frostbite.

Dry Needling

Dry needling, also known as myofascial trigger point dry needling, is an alternative medicine technique similar to acupuncture. Dry needling is sometimes also known as intramuscular stimulation (IMS). It involves the use of either solid filiform needles or hollow-core hypodermic needles for therapy of muscle pain, including pain related to myofascial pain syndrome. Dry needling is mainly used to treat myofascial trigger points, but it is also used to target connective tissue, neural ailments, and muscular ailments. The American Physical Therapy Association defines dry needling as a technique used to treat dysfunction of skeletal muscle and connective tissue, minimize peripheral nociception (pain), and improve or regulate structural or functional damage.

The efficacy of dry needling as a treatment for muscle pain is still not ascertained and there remains no scientific consensus whether it is effective. Some results suggest that it is an effective treatment for certain kinds of muscle pain, while other studies have shown no benefit compared to a placebo. Currently, dry needling is being practiced in the United States, Europe, Australia, and other countries; however, not enough high-quality, long-term, and large-scale studies have been done on the technique to draw clear conclusions about its efficacy.

The origin of the term “dry needling” is attributed to Janet G. Travell. However, Travell did not elaborate on the details on the techniques of dry needling; the current techniques of dry needling were based on the traditional and western medical acupuncture. The two techniques Travell described are the injection of a local anesthetic and the mechanical use of a hypodermic needle without injecting a solution. Travell preferred a 22-gauge, 1.5-in hypodermic needle for trigger point therapy and used this needle for both injection therapy and dry needling. Travell never used an acupuncture needle. Travell had access to acupuncture needles but reasoned that they were far too thin for trigger point therapy. She preferred hypodermic needles because of their strength and tactile feedback: "A 22-gauge, 3.8-cm (1.5-in) needle is usually suitable for most superficial muscles. In hyperalgesic patients, a 25-gauge, 3.8-cm (1.5-in) needle may cause less discomfort, but will not provide the clear "feel" of the structures being penetrated by the needle and is more likely to be deflected by the dense contraction knots that are the target A 27-gauge needle, 3.8-cm (1.5-in) needle is even more flexible; the tip is more likely to be deflected by the contraction knots and it provides less tactile feedback for precision injection".

Although dry needling originally utilized only hypodermic needles due to the concern that solid needles had neither the strength or tactile feedback that hypodermic needles provided and that the needle could be deflected by "dense contraction knots", those concerns have proven unfounded and many healthcare practitioners who perform dry needling have found that the acupuncture needles not only provides better tactile feedback but also penetrate the "dense muscle knots" better and are easier to manage and caused less discomfort to patients. For that reason, both the use of hypodermic needles and the use of acupuncture needles are now accepted in dry needling practices. Ofttimes practitioners who use hypodermic needles also provide trigger point injection treatment to patients and therefore find the use of hypodermic needles a better choice. As their use became more common, some dry needling practitioners without acupuncture in their scope of practice, started to refer to these needles by their technical design term as "solid filiform needles" as opposed to the FDA designation "acupuncture needle."

The "solid filiform needle" used in dry needling is regulated by the FDA as a Class II medical device described in the code titled. Per the Food and Drug Act of 1906 and the subsequent amendments to said act, the FDA definition applies to how the needles can be marketed and does not mean that acupuncture is the only medical procedure where these needles can be used. Dry needling using such a needle contrasts with the use of a hollow hypodermic needle to inject substances such as saline solution, botox or corticosteroids to the same point.

Dry needling for the treatment of myofascial (muscular) trigger points is based on theories similar, but not exclusive, to traditional acupuncture; both acupuncture and dry needling target the trigger points, which is a direct and palpable source of patient pain. A high degree of correspondence is reported between myofascial trigger point dry needling and traditional western acupuncture. Acupuncture and dry needling are similar in the underlying phenomenon and neural processes between trigger points and acupuncture points. There is a high degree of correspondence between published locations of trigger points and classical acupuncture points for the relief of pain. Dry needling, and its treatment techniques and desired effects, would be most directly comparable to the use of 'a-shi' points in acupuncture. However, dry needling theory only begins to describe the complex sensation referral patterns that have been documented as "channels" or "meridians" in Chinese Medicine. What further distinguishes dry needling from traditional acupuncture is that it does not use the full range of traditional theories of Chinese Medicine which is used to treat not only pain, but also other non-musculoskeletal issues that often cause pain. The distinction between trigger points and acupuncture points for the relief of pain is blurred.

The debated distinction between dry needling and acupuncture has become a controversy because it relates to an issue of scope of practice of various professions. Acupuncturists claim that dry needling is a form of acupuncture that doesn't fall in the scope of physical therapists, chiropractors, or the majority of other healthcare professionals; whereas those healthcare professionals claim dry needling is not acupuncture, but rather a procedure that is rooted in biomedical modern sciences. To become a certified acupuncturist requires hundred of hours spent in educational programs, national level exams, and good professional standings. On the other hand, to be certified in dry needling requires continued education or a certification program that is not yet regulated with strict standards; in addition, there is a general lack of policymakers, evaluation systems, or healthcare standards governing the technique of dry needling.

Technique

Technique for dry needling depends on which tissue is being targeted and what the overall objective of the treatment is. For example, one of the most common treatment objectives for dry needling, myofascial trigger points (TrPs), differs physiologically from treatments for scar tissue, connective tissue issues, and other medical issues.

In the treatment of trigger points for persons with myofascial pain syndrome, dry needling is an invasive procedure in which a filiform needle is inserted into the skin and muscle directly at a myofascial trigger point. A myofascial trigger point consists of multiple, hyperirritable contraction knots related to the production and maintenance of the pain cycle; essentially, myofascial trigger points will generate much local pain upon stimulation or irritation. Deep dry needling for treating trigger points was first introduced by Czech physician Karel Lewit in 1979. Lewit had noticed that the success of injections into trigger points in relieving pain was apparently unconnected to the analgesic used.

Dry needling can be divided into categories in terms of depth of penetration: deep and superficial dry needling. Deep dry needling will inactivate myofascial triggers points by provoking a local twitch response (LTR), which is an involuntary spinal cord reflex in which the muscle fibers in the taut band of muscle contract. The LTR indicates the proper placement of the needle in a trigger point. Dry needling that elicits LTRs improves treatment outcomes, and may work by activating endogenous opioids. The activation of the endogenous opioids is for an analgesic effect using the Gate Control Theory of Pain. In addition to relieving myofascial trigger points, deep dry needling is also identified to decreases pain, increase range of motion, and minimize myofascial trigger point irritability. In regards to the factor of pain reduction, relief occurs at four central levels: local pain, spinal pain through nerves, brain stem pain, and higher brain center pain.

The relief of myofascial trigger points has been more highly researched than relief of connective tissues, muscle fascia, muscle tension, and scar tissue; however, the American Physical Therapy Association claims that there potentially may be some benefits of dry needling on these ailments according to some available evidence. The APTA also disclaims that dry needling should not be used as a standalone procedure, but should be used in conjunction with other treatment methods, including manual soft tissue mobilization, neuromuscular re-education, functional retraining, and therapeutic exercises. Once the needle is inserted, one can manually or electrically stimulate the filiform needle depending for the desired effect of treatment.

Efficacy

There is currently no standardized form of dry needling. There is a general scarcity of extensive research in the field. Many studies published about dry needling are not randomized, contain small sample sizes, and have high dropout rates. A review recommended the usage of dry needling, compared to sham or placebo, for decreasing pain immediately after treatment and at 4 weeks in patients with upper quarter myofascial pain syndrome. However, the authors caution that "the limited number of studies performed to date, combined with methodological flaws in many of the studies, prompts caution in interpreting the results of the meta-analysis performed". Similarly, a second review of dry needling found insufficient high-quality evidence for the use of direct dry needling for short and long-term pain and disability reduction in patients with musculoskeletal pain syndromes. The same review reported that robust evidence validating the clinical diagnostic criteria for trigger point identification or diagnosis is lacking and that high-quality studies demonstrate that manual examination for the identification and localization of a trigger point is neither valid nor reliable between-examiners.

Three more recent reviews reached similar conclusions: little evidence supporting the use of trigger point dry needling to treat upper shoulder pain and dysfunction, evidence not robust enough to draw a clear conclusion about safety and efficacy, and that dry needling for the treatment of myofascial pain syndrome in the lower back appeared to be a useful addition to standard therapies, but stated clear recommendations could not be made because the published studies were small and of low quality.

Chiropractic

Chiropractic is a pseudoscientific complementary and alternative medicine (CAM) that is concerned with the diagnosis and treatment of mechanical disorders of the musculoskeletal system, especially the spine. Chiropractors have proposed, especially those in the field's early history, that such disorders affect general health via the nervous system. The main chiropractic treatment technique involves manual therapy, especially manipulation of the spine, other joints, and soft tissues, but may also include exercises and health and lifestyle counseling. Chiropractors are not physicians or medical doctors.

Reviews of controlled clinical studies of treatments used by chiropractors have not found evidence that chiropractic manipulation is effective, with the possible exception of treatment for back pain. A critical evaluation found that collectively, spinal manipulation was ineffective at treating any condition. Spinal manipulation may be cost-effective for sub-acute or chronic low back pain but the results for acute low back pain were insufficient. The efficacy and cost-effectiveness of maintenance chiropractic care are unknown. There is not sufficient data to establish the safety of chiropractic manipulations. It is frequently associated with mild to moderate adverse effects, with serious or fatal complications in rare cases. There is controversy regarding the degree of risk of vertebral artery dissection, which can lead to stroke and death, from cervical manipulation. Several deaths have been associated with this technique and it has been suggested that the relationship is causative, a claim which is disputed by many chiropractors.

Chiropractic is well established in the United States, Canada, and Australia. It overlaps with other manual-therapy professions such as osteopathy and physical therapy. Most who seek chiropractic care do so for low back pain. Back and neck pain are considered the specialties of chiropractic, but many chiropractors treat ailments other than musculoskeletal issues. Many chiropractors describe themselves as primary care providers, but the chiropractic clinical training does not support the requirements to be considered primary care providers. Chiropractic has two main groups: "straights", now the minority, emphasize vitalism, "innate intelligence", and consider vertebral subluxations to be the cause of all disease; "mixers", the majority, are more open to mainstream views and conventional medical techniques, such as exercise, massage, and ice therapy.

Chiropractic is generally categorized as complementary and alternative medicine (CAM), which focuses on manipulation of the musculoskeletal system, especially the spine. Its founder, D.D. Palmer, called it "a science of healing without drugs".

Chiropractic's origins lie in the folk medicine of bonesetting, and as it evolved it incorporated vitalism, spiritual inspiration and rationalism. Its early philosophy was based on deduction from irrefutable doctrine, which helped distinguish chiropractic from medicine, provided it with legal and political defenses against claims of practicing medicine without a license, and allowed chiropractors to establish themselves as an autonomous profession. This "straight" philosophy, taught to generations of chiropractors, rejects the inferential reasoning of the scientific method, and relies on deductions from vitalistic first principles rather than on the materialism of science. However, most practitioners tend to incorporate scientific research into chiropractic, and most practitioners are "mixers" who attempt to combine the materialistic reductionism of science with the metaphysics of their predecessors and with the holistic paradigm of wellness. A 2008 commentary proposed that chiropractic actively divorce itself from the straight philosophy as part of a campaign to eliminate untestable dogma and engage in critical thinking and evidence-based research.

Two chiropractic belief system constructs	
The testable principle	The untestable metaphor
Chiropractic adjustment ↓ Restoration of structural integrity ↓ Improvement of health status	Universal intelligence ↓ Innate intelligence ↓ Body physiology
Materialistic	Vitalistic
• Operational definitions possible. • Lends itself to scientific inquiry.	• Origin of holism in chiropractic. • Cannot be proven or disproven.

Although a wide diversity of ideas exist among chiropractors, they share the belief that the spine and health are related in a fundamental way, and that this relationship is mediated through the nervous system. Some chiropractors claim spinal manipulation can have an effect on a variety of ailments such as irritable bowel syndrome and asthma.

Chiropractic philosophy includes the following perspectives:

Holism assumes that health is affected by everything in an individual's environment; some sources also include a spiritual or existential dimension. In contrast, reductionism in chiropractic reduces causes and cures of health problems to a single factor, vertebral subluxation. Homeostasis emphasizes the body's inherent self-healing abilities. Chiropractic's early notion of innate intelligence can be thought of as a metaphor for homeostasis.

A large number of chiropractors fear that if they do not separate themselves from the traditional vitalistic concept of innate intelligence, chiropractic will continue to be seen as a fringe profession. A variant of chiropractic called naprapathy originated in Chicago in the early twentieth century. It holds that manual manipulation of soft tissue can reduce "interference" in the body and thus improve health.

Straights and Mixers

Table: Range of belief perspectives in chiropractic.

Perspective attribute	Potential belief endpoints	
Scope of practice:	narrow ("straight") ←	→ broad ("mixer")
Diagnostic approach:	intuitive ←	→ analytical

Philosophic orientation:	vitalistic ←	→ materialistic
Scientific orientation:	descriptive ←	→ experimental
Process orientation:	implicit ←	→ explicit
Practice attitude:	doctor/model-centered ←	→ patient/situation-centered
Professional integration:	separate and distinct ←	→ integrated into mainstream

Straight chiropractors adhere to the philosophical principles set forth by D.D. and B.J. Palmer, and retain metaphysical definitions and vitalistic qualities. Straight chiropractors believe that vertebral subluxation leads to interference with an "innate intelligence" exerted via the human nervous system and is a primary underlying risk factor for many diseases. Straights view the medical diagnosis of patient complaints, which they consider to be the "secondary effects" of subluxations, to be unnecessary for chiropractic treatment. Thus, straight chiropractors are concerned primarily with the detection and correction of vertebral subluxation via adjustment and do not "mix" other types of therapies into their practice style. Their philosophy and explanations are metaphysical in nature and they prefer to use traditional chiropractic lexicon terminology such as "perform spinal analysis", "detect subluxation", "correct with adjustment". They prefer to remain separate and distinct from mainstream health care. Although considered the minority group, "they have been able to transform their status as purists and heirs of the lineage into influence dramatically out of proportion to their numbers."

Mixer chiropractors "mix" diagnostic and treatment approaches from chiropractic, medical or osteopathic viewpoints and make up the majority of chiropractors. Unlike straight chiropractors, mixers believe subluxation is one of many causes of disease, and hence they tend to be open to mainstream medicine. Many of them incorporate mainstream medical diagnostics and employ conventional treatments including techniques of physical therapy such as exercise, stretching, massage, ice packs, electrical muscle stimulation, therapeutic ultrasound, and moist heat. Some mixers also use techniques from alternative medicine, including nutritional supplements, acupuncture, homeopathy, herbal remedies, and biofeedback.

Although mixers are the majority group, many of them retain belief in vertebral subluxation as shown in a 2003 survey of 1,100 North American chiropractors, which found that 88 percent wanted to retain the term "vertebral subluxation complex", and that when asked to estimate the percent of disorders of internal organs that subluxation significantly contributes to, the mean response was 62 percent. A 2008 survey of 6,000 American chiropractors demonstrated that most chiropractors seem to believe that a subluxation-based clinical approach may be of limited utility for addressing visceral disorders, and greatly favored non-subluxation-based clinical approaches for such conditions. The same survey showed that most chiropractors generally believed that the majority of their clinical approach for addressing musculoskeletal/biomechanical disorders such as back pain was based on subluxation. Chiropractors often offer conventional therapies such as physical therapy and lifestyle counseling, and it may for the lay person be difficult to distinguish the unscientific from the scientific.

Vertebral Subluxation

Palmer hypothesized that vertebral joint misalignments, which he termed *vertebral subluxations*, interfered with the body's function and its inborn ability to heal itself. D. D. Palmer repudiated his earlier theory that vertebral subluxations caused pinched nerves in the intervertebral spaces in favor of subluxations causing altered nerve vibration, either too tense or too slack, affecting the tone (health) of the end organ. D. D. Palmer, using a vitalistic approach, imbued the term *subluxation* with a metaphysical and philosophical meaning. He qualified this by noting that knowledge of innate intelligence was not essential to the competent practice of chiropractic. This concept was later expanded upon by his son, B. J. Palmer, and was instrumental in providing the legal basis of differentiating chiropractic from conventional medicine. In 1910, D. D. Palmer theorized that the nervous system controlled health:

"Physiologists divide nerve-fibers, which form the nerves, into two classes, afferent and efferent. Impressions are made on the peripheral afferent fiber-endings; these create sensations that are transmitted to the center of the nervous system. Efferent nerve-fibers carry impulses out from the center to their endings. Most of these go to muscles and are therefore called motor impulses; some are secretory and enter glands; a portion are inhibitory, their function being to restrain secretion. Thus, nerves carry impulses outward and sensations inward. The activity of these nerves, or rather their fibers, may become excited or allayed by impingement, the result being a modification of functionality – too much or not enough action – which is disease."

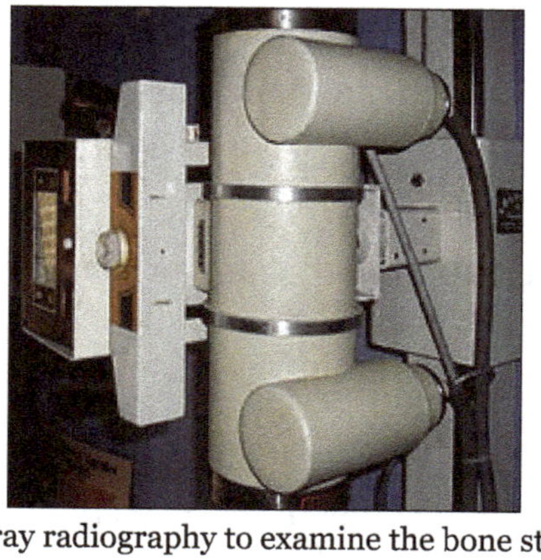

Chiropractors use x-ray radiography to examine the bone structure of a patient.

Vertebral subluxation, a core concept of traditional chiropractic, remains unsubstantiated and largely untested, and a debate about whether to keep it in the chiropractic paradigm has been ongoing for decades. In general, critics of traditional subluxation-based chiropractic (including chiropractors) are skeptical of its clinical value, dogmatic beliefs and metaphysical approach. While straight chiropractic still retains the traditional vitalistic construct espoused by the founders, evidence-based chiropractic suggests that a mechanistic view will allow chiropractic care to become integrated into the wider health care community. This is still a continuing source of debate within the chiropractic profession as well, with some schools of chiropractic still teaching the traditional/straight subluxation-based chiropractic, while others have moved towards an evidence-based chiropractic that rejects metaphysical foundings and limits itself to primarily neuromusculoskeletal conditions.

In 2005, the chiropractic subluxation was defined by the World Health Organization as "a lesion or dysfunction in a joint or motion segment in which alignment, movement integrity and/or physiological function are altered, although contact between joint surfaces remains intact. It is essentially a functional entity, which may influence biomechanical and neural integrity." This differs from the medical definition of subluxation as a significant structural displacement, which can be seen with static imaging techniques such as X-rays. This exposes patients to harmful ionizing radiation for no evidentially supported reason. The 2008 book *Trick or Treatment* states "X-rays can reveal neither the subluxations nor the innate intelligence associated with chiropractic philosophy, because they do not exist." Attorney David Chapman-Smith, Secretary-General of the World Federation of Chiropractic, has stated that "Medical critics have asked how there can be a subluxation if it cannot be seen on X-ray. The answer is that the chiropractic subluxation is essentially a functional entity, not structural, and is therefore no more visible on static X-ray than a limp or headache or any other functional problem." The General Chiropractic Council, the statutory regulatory body for chiropractors in the United Kingdom, states that the chiropractic vertebral subluxation complex "is not supported by any clinical research evidence that would allow claims to be made that it is the cause of disease."

As of 2014, the National Board of Chiropractic Examiners states "The specific focus of chiropractic practice is known as the chiropractic subluxation or joint dysfunction. A subluxation is a health concern that manifests in the skeletal joints, and, through complex anatomical and physiological relationships, affects the nervous system and may lead to reduced function, disability or illness."

Scope of Practice

Chiropractors emphasize the conservative management of the neuromusculoskeletal system without the use of medicines or surgery, with special emphasis on the spine. Back and neck pain are the specialties of chiropractic but many chiropractors treat ailments other than musculoskeletal issues. There is a range of opinions among chiropractors: some believed that treatment should be confined to the spine, or back and neck pain; others disagreed. For example, while one 2009 survey of American chiropractors had found that 73% classified themselves as "back pain/musculoskeletal specialists", the label "back and neck pain specialists" was regarded by 47% of them as a *least* desirable description in a 2005 international survey. Chiropractic combines aspects from mainstream and alternative medicine, and there is no agreement about how to define the profession: although chiropractors have many attributes of primary care providers, chiropractic has more attributes of a medical specialty like dentistry or podiatry. It has been proposed that chiropractors specialize in nonsurgical spine care, instead of attempting to also treat other problems, but the more expansive view of chiropractic is still widespread.

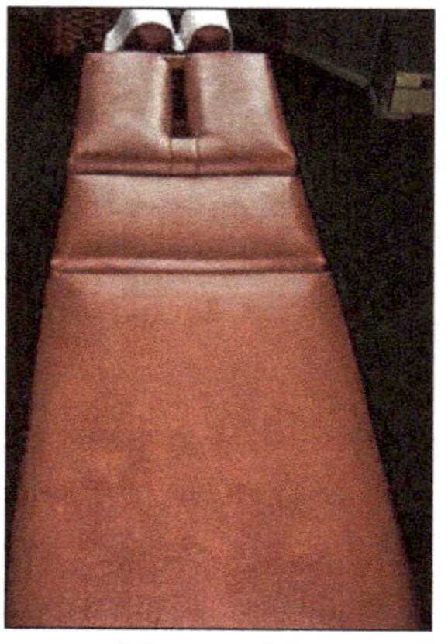

A treatment table at a chiropractic office.

Mainstream health care and governmental organizations such as the World Health Organization consider chiropractic to be complementary and alternative medicine (CAM); and a 2008 study reported that 31% of surveyed chiropractors categorized chiropractic as CAM, 27% as integrated medicine, and 12% as mainstream medicine. Many chiropractors believe they are primary care providers, including US and UK chiropractors, but the length, breadth, and depth of chiropractic clinical training do not support the requirements to be considered primary care providers, so their role on primary care is limited and disputed.

Chiropractic overlaps with several other forms of manual therapy, including massage therapy, osteopathy, physical therapy, and sports medicine. Chiropractic is autonomous from and competitive with mainstream medicine, and osteopathy outside the US remains primarily a manual medical system; physical therapists work alongside and cooperate with mainstream medicine, and osteopathic medicine in the U.S. has merged with the medical profession. Practitioners may distinguish these competing approaches through claims that, compared to other therapists, chiropractors heavily emphasize spinal manipulation, tend to use firmer manipulative techniques, and promote maintenance care; that osteopaths use a wider variety of treatment procedures; and that physical therapists emphasize machinery and exercise.

Chiropractic diagnosis may involve a range of methods including skeletal imaging, observational and tactile assessments, and orthopedic and neurological evaluation. A chiropractor may also refer a patient to an appropriate specialist, or co-manage with another health care provider. Common patient management involves spinal manipulation

(SM) and other manual therapies to the joints and soft tissues, rehabilitative exercises, health promotion, electrical modalities, complementary procedures, and lifestyle advice.

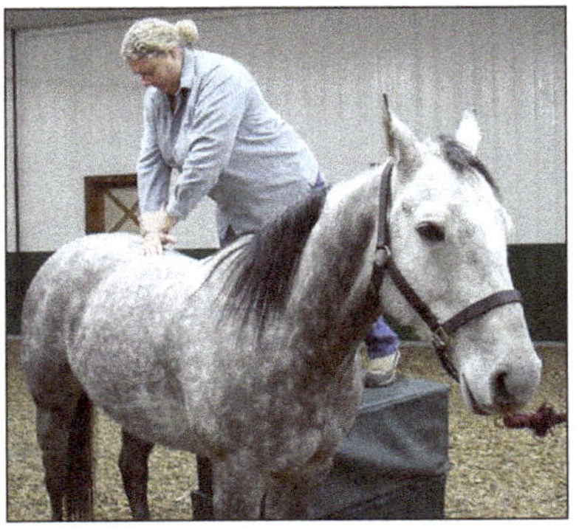

A chiropractic adjustment of a horse.

Chiropractors are not normally licensed to write medical prescriptions or perform major surgery in the United States, (although New Mexico has become the first US state to allow "advanced practice" trained chiropractors to prescribe certain medications.). In the US, their scope of practice varies by state, based on inconsistent views of chiropractic care: some states, such as Iowa, broadly allow treatment of "human ailments"; some, such as Delaware, use vague concepts such as "transition of nerve energy" to define scope of practice; others, such as New Jersey, specify a severely narrowed scope. US states also differ over whether chiropractors may conduct laboratory tests or diagnostic procedures, dispense dietary supplements, or use other therapies such as homeopathy and acupuncture; in Oregon they can become certified to perform minor surgery and to deliver children via natural childbirth. A 2003 survey of North American chiropractors found that a slight majority favored allowing them to write prescriptions for over-the-counter drugs. A survey found that 72% of Swiss chiropractors considered their ability to prescribe nonprescription medication as an advantage for chiropractic treatment.

A related field, veterinary chiropractic, applies manual therapies to animals and is recognized in 40 US states, but is not recognized by the American Chiropractic Association as being chiropractic. It remains controversial within certain segments of the veterinary, and chiropractic profession.

No single profession "owns" spinal manipulation and there is little consensus as to which profession should administer SM, raising concerns by chiropractors that other medical physicians could "steal" SM procedures from chiropractors. A focus on evidence-based SM research has also raised concerns that the resulting practice guidelines could limit the scope of chiropractic practice to treating backs and necks. Two U.S. states prohibit physical therapists from performing SM, some states allow them to do it only if they have completed advanced training in SM, and some states allow only chiropractors to perform SM, or only chiropractors and physicians. Bills to further prohibit non-chiropractors from performing SM are regularly introduced into state legislatures and are opposed by physical therapist organizations.

Treatments

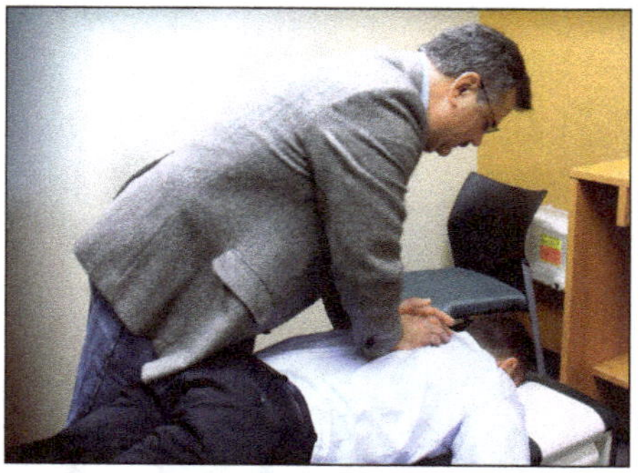

A chiropractor performs an adjustment on a patient.

Spinal manipulation, which chiropractors call "spinal adjustment" or "chiropractic adjustment", is the most common treatment used in chiropractic care. Spinal manipulation is a passive manual maneuver during which a three-joint complex is taken past the normal range of movement, but not so far as to dislocate or damage the joint. Its defining factor is a dynamic thrust, which is a sudden force that causes an audible release and attempts to increase a joint's range of motion. High-velocity, low-amplitude spinal manipulation (HVLA-SM) thrusts have physiological effects that signal neural discharge from paraspinal muscle tissues, depending on duration and amplitude of the thrust are factors of the degree in paraspinal muscle spindles activation. Clinical skill in employing HVLA-SM thrusts depends on the ability of the practitioner to handle the duration and magnitude of the load. More generally, spinal manipulative therapy (SMT) describes techniques where the hands are used to manipulate, massage, mobilize, adjust, stimulate, apply traction to, or otherwise influence the spine and related tissues.

There are several schools of chiropractic adjustive techniques, although most chiropractors mix techniques from several schools. The following adjustive procedures were received by more than 10% of patients of licensed U.S. chiropractors in a 2003 survey: Diversified technique (full-spine manipulation, employing various techniques), extremity adjusting, Activator technique (which uses a spring-loaded tool to deliver precise adjustments to the spine), Thompson Technique (which relies on a drop table and detailed procedural protocols), Gonstead (which emphasizes evaluating the spine along with specific adjustment that avoids rotational vectors), Cox/flexion-distraction (a gentle, low-force adjusting procedure which mixes chiropractic with osteopathic principles and utilizes specialized adjusting tables with movable parts), adjustive instrument, Sacro-Occipital Technique (which models the spine as a torsion bar), Nimmo Receptor-Tonus Technique, applied kinesiology (which emphasises "muscle testing" as a diagnostic tool), and cranial. Chiropractic biophysics technique uses inverse functions of rotations during spinal manipulation. Koren Specific Technique (KST) may use their hands, or they may use an electric device known as an "ArthroStim" for assessment and spinal manipulations. Insurers in the US and UK that cover other chiropractic techniques exclude KST from coverage because they consider it to be "experimental and investigational". Medicine-assisted manipulation, such as manipulation under anesthesia, involves sedation or local anesthetic and is done by a team that includes an anesthesiologist; a review did not find enough evidence to make recommendations about its use for chronic low back pain.

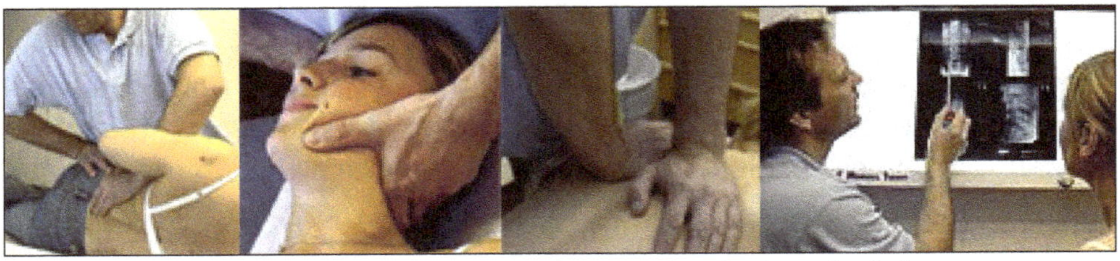

Lumbar, cervical and thoracic chiropractic spinal manipulation.

Many other procedures are used by chiropractors for treating the spine, other joints and tissues, and general health issues. The following procedures were received by more than one-third of patients of licensed U.S. chiropractors in a 2003 survey: Diversified technique, physical fitness/exercise promotion, corrective or therapeutic exercise, ergonomic/postural advice, self-care strategies, activities of daily living, changing risky/unhealthy behaviors, nutritional/dietary recommendations, relaxation/stress reduction recommendations, ice pack/cryotherapy, extremity adjusting, trigger point therapy, and disease prevention/early screening advice.

Effectiveness

There is no good evidence that chiropractic is effective for the treatment of any medical condition, except perhaps for certain kinds of back pain. Generally, the research carried out into the effectiveness of chiropractic has been of poor quality. Numerous controlled clinical studies of treatments used by chiropractors have been conducted, with varied results. Research published by chiropractors is distinctly biased. For reviews of SM for back pain chiropractic authors tend to have positive conclusions, while others did not show any effectiveness.

There is a wide range of ways to measure treatment outcomes. Chiropractic care, like all medical treatment, benefits from the placebo response. It is difficult to construct a trustworthy placebo for clinical trials of spinal manipulative therapy (SMT), as experts often disagree about whether a proposed placebo actually has no effect. The efficacy of maintenance care in chiropractic is unknown.

Available evidence covers the following conditions:

- Low back pain: A review found very low to moderate evidence that SMT was no more effective than inert interventions, sham SMT or as an adjunct therapy for acute low back pain. The same review found that SMT appears to be no better than other recommended therapies. A 2012 overview of systematic reviews found that collectively, SM failed to show it is an effective intervention for pain. A review found strong evidence that suggests there is no clinically meaningful difference between SMT and other treatments for reducing pain and improving function for chronic low back pain. A review found no current evidence to support or refute a clinically significant difference between the effects of combined chiropractic interventions and other interventions for chronic or mixed duration low back pain. A review found that most studies suggest SMT achieves equivalent or superior improvement in pain and function when compared with other commonly used interventions for short, intermediate, and long-term follow-up. Specific guidelines concerning the treatment of nonspecific (i.e., unknown cause) low back pain are inconsistent between countries.

- Radiculopathy: A review and meta-analysis found a statistically significant improvement in overall recovery from sciatica following SM, when compared to usual care, and suggested that SM may be considered. There is moderate quality evidence to support the use of SM for the treatment of acute lumbar radiculopathy and acute lumbar disc herniation with associated radiculopathy. There is low or very low evidence supporting SM for chronic lumbar spine-related extremity symptoms and cervical spine-related extremity symptoms of any duration and no evidence exists for the treatment of thoracic radiculopathy.
- Whiplash and other neck pain: There is no consensus on the effectiveness of manual therapies for neck pain. A review found that the data suggests that there are minimal short- and long-term treatment differences when comparing manipulation or mobilization of the cervical spine to physical therapy or exercise for neck pain improvement. A review found that although there is insufficient evidence that thoracic SM is more effective than other treatments, it is a suitable intervention to treat some patients with non-specific neck pain. A review found that thoracic SM may offer short-term improvement for the treatment of acute or subacute mechanical neck pain; although the body of literature is still weak. A review found low quality evidence that suggests cervical manipulation may offer better short-term pain relief than a control for neck pain, and moderate evidence that cervical manipulation and mobilization produced similar effects on pain, function and patient satisfaction. A review found low level evidence that suggests chiropractic care improves cervical range of motion and pain in the management of whiplash.
- Headache: A review found evidence that suggests that chiropractic SMT might be as effective as propranolol or topiramate in the prevention of migraine headaches. A review found evidence that does not support the use of SM for the treatment of migraine headaches. A review found no rigorous evidence supporting SM or other manual therapies for tension headache. A review found that the evidence was weak for effectiveness of chiropractic manipulation for tension headache, and that it was probably more effective for tension headache than for migraine.

- Extremity conditions: A review and meta-analysis concluded that the addition of manual mobilizations to an exercise program for the treatment of knee osteoarthritis resulted in better pain relief than a supervised exercise program alone and suggested that manual therapists consider adding manual mobilization to optimize supervised active exercise programs. There is silver level evidence that manual therapy is more effective than exercise for the treatment of hip osteoarthritis, however this evidence could be considered to be inconclusive. There is a small amount of research into the efficacy of chiropractic treatment for upper limbs, limited to low level evidence supporting chiropractic management of shoulder pain and limited or fair evidence supporting chiropractic management of leg conditions.
- Other: A review found insufficient low bias evidence to support the use of spinal manipulation as a therapy for the treatment of hypertension. A review found moderate evidence to support the use of manual therapy for cervicogenic dizziness. There is very weak evidence for chiropractic care for adult scoliosis (curved or rotated spine) and no scientific data for idiopathic adolescent scoliosis. A review found that few studies of chiropractic care for nonmusculoskeletal conditions are available, and they are typically not of high quality; it also found that the entire clinical encounter of chiropractic care (as opposed to just SM) provides benefit to patients with cervicogenic dizziness, and that the evidence from reviews is negative, or too weak to draw conclusions, for a wide variety of other nonmusculoskeletal conditions, including ADHD/learning disabilities, dizziness, high blood pressure, and vision conditions. Other reviews have found no evidence of significant benefit for asthma, baby colic, bedwetting, carpal tunnel syndrome, fibromyalgia, gastrointestinal disorders, kinetic imbalance due to suboccipital strain (KISS) in infants, menstrual cramps, insomnia, postmenopausal symptoms, or pelvic and back pain during pregnancy. As there is no evidence of effectiveness or safety for cervical manipulation for baby colic, it is not endorsed.

Safety

The World Health Organization found chiropractic care in general is safe when employed skillfully and appropriately. There is not sufficient data to establish the safety of chiropractic manipulations. Manipulation is regarded as relatively safe but complications can arise, and it has known adverse effects, risks and contraindications. Absolute contraindications to spinal manipulative therapy are conditions that should not be manipulated; these contraindications include rheumatoid arthritis and conditions known to result in unstable joints. Relative contraindications are conditions where increased risk is acceptable in some situations and where low-force and soft-tissue techniques are treatments of choice; these contraindications include osteoporosis. Although most contraindications apply only to manipulation of the affected region, some neurological signs indicate referral to emergency medical services; these include sudden and severe headache or neck pain unlike that previously experienced. Indirect risks of chiropractic involve delayed or missed diagnoses through consulting a chiropractor.

Spinal manipulation is associated with frequent, mild and temporary adverse effects, including new or worsening pain or stiffness in the affected region. They have been estimated to occur in 33% to 61% of patients, and frequently occur within an hour of treatment and disappear within 24 to 48 hours; adverse reactions appear to be more common following manipulation than mobilization. The most frequently stated adverse effects are mild headache, soreness, and briefly elevated pain fatigue. Chiropractic is correlated with a very high incidence of minor adverse effects. Chiropractic are more commonly associated with serious related adverse effects than other professionals following manipulation. Rarely, spinal manipulation, particularly on the upper spine, can also result in complications that can lead to permanent disability or death; these can occur in adults and children. There is a case of a three-month-old dying following manipulation of the neck area. Estimates vary widely for the incidence of these complications, and the actual incidence is unknown, due to high levels of underreporting and to the difficulty of linking manipulation to adverse effects such as stroke, which is a particular concern. Adverse effects are poorly reported in recent studies investigating chiropractic manipulations. A review concludes that the level of reporting is unsuitable and unacceptable. Reports of serious adverse events have occurred, resulting from spinal manipulation therapy of the lumbopelvic region. Estimates for serious adverse events vary from 5 strokes per 100,000 manipulations to 1.46 serious adverse events per 10 million manipulations and 2.68 deaths per 10 million manipulations, though it was determined that there was inadequate data to be conclusive. Several case reports show temporal associations between interventions and potentially serious complications. The published medical literature contains reports of 26 deaths since 1934 following chiropractic manipulations and many more seem to remain unpublished.

Vertebrobasilar artery stroke (VAS) is statistically associated with chiropractic services in persons under 45 years of age, but it is similarly associated with general practitioner services, suggesting that these associations are likely explained by preexisting conditions. Weak to moderately strong evidence supports causation (as opposed to statistical association) between cervical manipulative therapy (CMT) and VAS. There is insufficient evidence to support a strong association or no association between cervical manipulation and stroke. While the biomechanical evidence is not sufficient to support the statement that CMT causes cervical artery dissection (CD), clinical reports suggest that mechanical forces have a part in a substantial number of CDs and the majority of population controlled studies found an association between CMT and VAS in young people. It is strongly recommended that practitioners consider the plausibility of CD as a symptom, and people can be informed of the association between CD and CMT before administrating manipulation of the cervical spine. There is controversy regarding the degree of risk of stroke from cervical manipulation. Many chiropractors state that, the association between chiropractic therapy and vertebral arterial dissection is not proven. However, it has been suggested that the causality between chiropractic cervical manipulation beyond the normal range of motion and vascular accidents is probable or definite. There is very low evidence supporting a small association between internal carotid artery dissection and chiropractic neck manipulation. The incidence of internal carotid artery dissection following cervical spine manipulation is unknown. The literature infrequently reports helpful data to better understand the association between cervical manipulative therapy, cervical artery dissection and stroke. The limited evidence is inconclusive that chiropractic spinal manipulation therapy is not a cause of intracranial hypotension. Cervical intradural disc herniation is very rare following spinal manipulation therapy.

Chiropractors, like other primary care providers, sometimes employ diagnostic imaging techniques such as X-rays and CT scans that rely on ionizing radiation. Although there is no clear evidence for the practice, some chiropractors may still X-ray a patient several times a year. Practice guidelines aim to reduce unnecessary radiation exposure, which increases cancer risk in proportion to the amount of radiation received. Research suggests that radiology instruction given at chiropractic schools worldwide seem to be evidence-based. Although, there seems to be a disparity between some schools and available evidence regarding the aspect of radiography for patients with acute low back pain without an indication of a serious disease, which may contribute to chiropractic overuse of radiography for low back pain.

Risk-benefit

A review concluded that no accurate assessment of risk-benefit exists for cervical manipulation. A review stated that there is no good evidence to assume that neck manipulation is an effective treatment for any medical condition and suggested a precautionary principle in healthcare for chiropractic intervention even if a causality with vertebral artery dissection after neck manipulation were merely a remote possibility. The same review concluded that the risk of death from manipulations to the neck outweighs the benefits. Chiropractors have criticized this conclusion, claiming that the author did not evaluate the potential benefits of spinal manipulation. Edzard Ernst stated "This detail was not the subject of my review. However, refer to such evaluations and should add that a report recently commissioned by the General Chiropractic Council did not support many of the outlandish claims made by many chiropractors across the world."

A review evaluating maintenance chiropractic care found that spinal manipulation is routinely associated with considerable harm and no compelling evidence exists to indicate that it adequately prevents symptoms or diseases, thus the risk-benefit is not evidently favorable.

Cost-effectiveness

A review suggested that the use of spine manipulation in clinical practice is a cost-effective treatment when used alone or in combination with other treatment approaches. A review found evidence supporting the cost-effectiveness of using spinal manipulation for the treatment of sub-acute or chronic low back pain; the results for acute low back pain were insufficient.

A review found that the reported cost-effectiveness of spinal manipulation in the United Kingdom compared favorably with other treatments for back pain, but that reports were based on data from clinical trials without sham controls and that the specific cost-effectiveness of the treatment (as opposed to non-specific effects) remains uncertain. A systematic review of economic evaluations of conservative treatments for low back pain found that significant quality problems in available studies meant that definite conclusions could not be drawn about the most cost-effective intervention. The cost-effectiveness of maintenance chiropractic care is unknown.

Analysis of a clinical and cost utilization data from the years 2003 to 2005 by an integrative medicine independent physician association (IPA) which looked the chiropractic services utilization found that the clinical and cost utilization of chiropractic services based on 70,274 member-months over a 7-year period decreased patient costs associate with the following use of services by 60% for in-hospital admissions, 59% for hospital days, 62% for outpatient surgeries and procedures, and 85% for pharmaceutical costs when compared with conventional medicine (visit to a medical doctor primary care provider) IPA performance for the same health maintenance organization product in the same geography and time frame.

Aquatic Therapy

Aquatic therapy refers to treatments and exercises performed in water for relaxation, fitness, physical rehabilitation, and other therapeutic benefit. Typically a qualified aquatic therapist gives constant attendance to a person receiving treatment in a heated therapy pool. Aquatic therapy techniques include Ai Chi, Aqua Running, Bad Ragaz Ring Method, Burdenko Method, Halliwick, Watsu, and other aquatic bodywork forms. Therapeutic applications include neurological disorders, spine pain, musculoskeletal pain, postoperative orthopedic rehabilitation, pediatric disabilities, and pressure ulcers.

Aquatic therapy refers to water-based treatments or exercises of therapeutic intent, in particular for relaxation, fitness, and physical rehabilitation. Treatments and exercises are performed while floating, partially submerged, or fully submerged in water. Many aquatic therapy procedures require constant attendance by a trained therapist, and are performed in a specialized temperature-controlled pool. Rehabilitation commonly focuses on improving the physical function associated with illness, injury, or disability.

Aquatic therapy encompasses a broad set of approaches and techniques, including aquatic exercise, physical therapy, aquatic bodywork, and other movement-based therapy in water (hydrokinesiotherapy). Treatment may be passive, involving a therapist or giver and a patient or receiver, or active, involving self-generated body positions, movement, or exercise. Examples include Halliwick Aquatic Therapy, Bad Ragaz Ring Method, Watsu, and Ai chi.

For orthopedic rehabilitation, aquatic therapy is considered to be synonymous with therapeutic aquatic exercise, aqua therapy, aquatic rehabilitation, water therapy, and pool therapy. Aquatic therapy can support restoration of function for many areas of orthopedics, including sports medicine, work conditioning, joint arthroplasty, and back rehabilitation programs. A strong aquatic component is especially beneficial for therapy programs where limited or non-weight bearing is desirable and where normal functioning is limited by inflammation, pain, guarding, muscle spasm, and limited range of motion (ROM). Water provides a controllable environment for reeducation of weak muscles and skill development for neurological and neuromuscular impairment, acute orthopedic or neuromuscular injury, rheumatological disease, or recovery from recent surgery.

Various properties of water contribute to therapeutic effects, including the ability to use water for resistance in place of gravity or weights; thermal stability that permits maintenance of near-constant temperature; hydrostatic pressure that supports and stabilizes, and that influences heart and lung function; buoyancy that permits flotation and reduces the effects of gravity; and turbulence and wave propagation that allow gentle manipulation and movement.

Techniques

Techniques for aquatic therapy include the following:

- Ai Chi: Ai Chi, developed in 1993 by Jun Konno, uses diaphragmatic breathing and active progressive resistance training in water to relax and strengthen the body, based on elements of qigong and Tai chi chuan.
- Aqua running: Aqua running (Deep Water Running or Aquajogging) is a form of cardiovascular conditioning, involving running or jogging in water, useful for injured athletes and those who desire a low-impact aerobic workout. Aqua running is performed in deep water using a floatation device (vest or belt) to support the head above water.
- Bad Ragaz Ring Method: The Bad Ragaz Ring Method (BRRM) focuses on rehabilitation of neuromuscular function using patterns of therapist-assisted exercise performed while the patient lies horizontal in water, with support provided by rings or floats around the neck, arms, pelvis, and knees. BRRM is an aquatic version of Proprioceptive Neuromuscular Facilitation (PNF) developed by physiotherapists at Bad Ragaz, Switzerland, as a synthesis of aquatic exercises designed by a German physician in the 1930s and land-based PNF developed by American physiotherapists in the 1950s and 1960s.

- Burdenko Method: The Burdenko Method, originally developed by Soviet professor of sports medicine Igor Burdenko, is an integrated land-water therapy approach that develops balance, coordination, flexibility, endurance, speed, and strength using the same methods as professional athletes. The water-based therapy uses buoyant equipment to challenge the center of buoyancy in vertical positions, exercising with movement in multiple directions, and at multiple speeds ranging from slow to fast.
- Halliwick Concept: The Halliwick Concept, originally developed by fluid mechanics engineer James McMillan in the late 1940s and 1950s at the Halliwick School for Girls with Disabilities in London, focuses on biophysical principles of motor control in water, in particular developing sense of balance (equilibrioception) and core stability. The Halliwick Ten-Point-Program implements the concept in a progressive program of mental adjustment, disengagement, and development of motor control, with an emphasis on rotational control, and applies the program to teach physically disabled people balance control, swimming, and independence. Halliwick Aquatic Therapy (also known as Water Specific Therapy, WST), implements the concept in patient-specific aquatic therapy.
- Watsu: Watsu is a form of aquatic bodywork, originally developed in the early 1980s by Harold Dull at Harbin Hot Springs, California, in which an aquatic therapist continuously supports and guides the person receiving treatment through a series of flowing movements and stretches that induce deep relaxation and provide therapeutic benefit. In the late 1980s and early 1990s physiotherapists began to use Watsu for a wide range of orthopedic and neurologic conditions, and to adapt the techniques for use with injury and disability.

Applications and Effectiveness

Applications of aquatic therapy include neurological disorders, spine pain, musculoskeletal pain, postoperative orthopedic rehabilitation, pediatric disabilities, and pressure ulcers.

A review of effects of aquatic interventions in children with neuromotor impairments found "substantial lack of evidence-based research evaluating the specific effects of aquatic interventions in this population".

For musculoskeletal rehabilitation, aquatic therapy is typically used to treat acute injuries as well as subjective pain of chronic conditions, such as arthritis. Water immersion has compressive effects and reflexively regulates blood vessel tone. Muscle blood flow increases by about 225% during immersion, as increased cardiac output is distributed to skin and muscle tissue. Flotation is able to counteract the effects of gravitational force on joints, creating a low impact environment for joints to perform within. The temperature changes, increase in systolic blood pressure to extremities, and overall increase in ambulation are factors which help immersion to alleviate pain. Aquatic

Therapy helps with pain and stiffness, but can also improve quality of life, tone the muscles in the body, and can help with movement in the knees and hips. Not only does aquatic therapy help with pain, but can benefit postural stability, meaning it can help to strengthen balance functions especially with people who have neurological disorders.

From a cardiopulmonary standpoint, aquatic therapy is often used because its effects mirror land-based effects but at lower speeds. During immersion, blood is displaced upwards into heart and there is an increase in pulse pressure due to increased cardiac filling. Cardiac volume increases 27-30%. Oxygen consumption is increased with exercise, and heart rate is increased at higher temperatures, and decreased at lower temperatures. However, immersion can worsen effects in cases of valvular insufficiency due to this cardiac and stroke volume increase. The aquatic environment is also not recommended for those who experience severe or uncontrolled heart failure.

Hydrotherapy

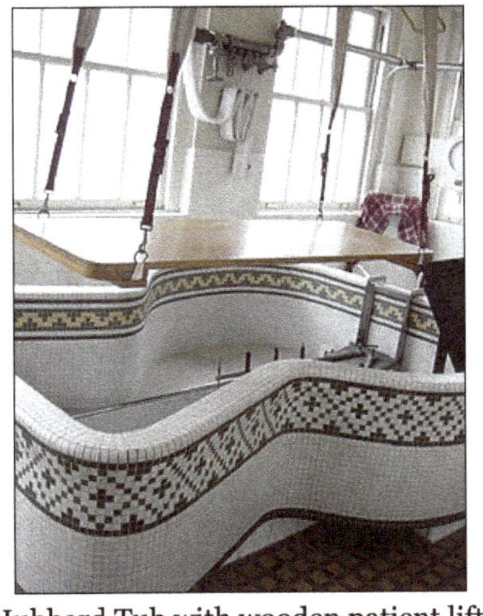

Hubbard Tub with wooden patient lift.

Hydrotherapy, formerly called hydropathy and also called water cure, is a part of alternative medicine (particularly naturopathy), occupational therapy, and physiotherapy, that involves the use of water for pain relief and treatment. The term encompasses a broad range of approaches and therapeutic methods that take advantage of the physical properties of water, such as temperature and pressure, for therapeutic purposes, to stimulate blood circulation and treat the symptoms of certain diseases.

Various therapies used in the present-day hydrotherapy employ water jets, underwater massage and mineral baths (e.g. balneotherapy, Iodine-Grine therapy, Kneipp treatments, Scotch hose, Swiss shower, thalassotherapy) or whirlpool bath, hot Roman bath, hot tub, Jacuzzi, cold plunge and mineral bath.

Uses

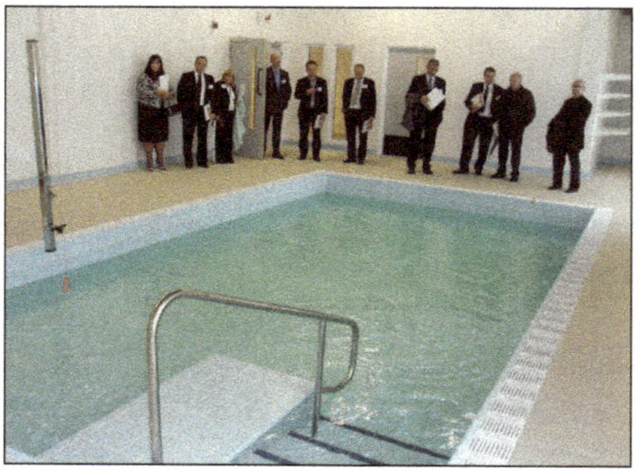

Hydrotherapy Pool.

Water therapy may be restricted to use as aquatic therapy, a form of physical therapy, and as a cleansing agent. However, it is also used as a medium for delivery of heat and cold to the body, which has long been the basis for its application. Hydrotherapy involves a range of methods and techniques, many of which use water as a medium to facilitate thermoregulatory reactions for therapeutic benefit.

Hydrotherapy is used as an adjunct to therapy, including in nursing, where its use is now long established. It continues to be widely used for burn treatment, although shower-based hydrotherapy techniques have been increasingly used in preference to full-immersion methods, partly for the ease of cleaning the equipment and reducing infections due to contamination. When removal of tissue is necessary for the treatment of wounds, hydrotherapy which performs selective mechanical debridement can be used. Examples of this include directed wound irrigation and therapeutic irrigation with suction.

Technique

The appliances and arrangements by means of which heat and cold are brought to bear are (a) packings, hot and cold, general and local, sweating and cooling; (b) hot air and steam baths; (c) general baths, of hot water and cold; (d) sitz (sitting), spinal, head and foot baths; (e) bandages (or compresses), wet and dry; also (f) fomentations and poultices, hot and cold, sinapisms, stupes, rubbings and water potations, hot and cold.

Hydrotherapy which involves submerging all or part of the body in water can involve several types of equipment:

- Full body immersion tanks (a "Hubbard tank" is a large size).
- Arm, hip, and leg whirlpool.

Whirling water movement, provided by mechanical pumps, has been used in water tanks since at least the 1940s. Similar technologies have been marketed for recreational use under the terms "hot tub" or "spa".

In some cases baths with whirlpool water flow aren't used to manage wounds because a whirlpool will not selectively target the tissue to be removed and can damage all tissue. Whirlpools also create an unwanted risk of bacterial infection, can damage fragile body tissue, and in the case of treating arms and legs, bring risk of complications from edema.

Telerehabilitation

Telerehabilitation (or e-rehabilitation) is the delivery of rehabilitation services over telecommunication networks and the internet. Most types of services fall into two categories: clinical assessment (the patient's functional abilities in his or her environment), and clinical therapy. Some fields of rehabilitation practice that have explored telerehabilitation are: neuropsychology, speech-language pathology, audiology, occupational therapy, and physical therapy. Telerehabilitation can deliver therapy to people who cannot travel to a clinic because the patient has a disability or because of travel time. Telerehabilitation also allows experts in rehabilitation to engage in a clinical consultation at a distance.

Most telerehabilitation is highly visual. As of 2006 the most commonly used modalities are via webcams, videoconferencing, phone lines, videophones and webpages containing rich Internet applications. The visual nature of telerehabilitation technology limits the types of rehabilitation services that can be provided. It is most widely used for neuropsychological rehabilitation; fitting of rehabilitation equipment such as wheelchairs, braces or artificial limbs; and in speech-language pathology. Rich internet applications for neuropsychological rehabilitation (aka cognitive rehabilitation) of cognitive impairment (from many etiologies) was first introduced in 2001. This endeavor has recently expanded as a teletherapy application for cognitive skills enhancement programs for school children. Tele-audiology (hearing assessments) is a growing application. As of 2006, telerehabilitation in the practice of occupational therapy and physical therapy are very limited, perhaps because these two disciplines are more "hands on".

Two important areas of telerehabilitation research are (1) demonstrating equivalence of assessment and therapy to in-person assessment and therapy, and (2) building new data collection systems to digitize information that a therapist can use in practice. Ground-breaking research in telehaptics (the sense of touch) and virtual reality may broaden the scope of telerehabilitation practice, in the future.

In the United States, the National Institute on Disability and Rehabilitation Research's (NIDRR) supports research and the development of telerehabilitation. NIDRR's grantees include the "Rehabilitation Engineering and Research Center" (RERC) at the University of Pittsburgh, the Rehabilitation Institute of Chicago, the State University of New York at Buffalo, and the National Rehabilitation Hospital in Washington DC. Other federal funders of research are the Veterans Administration, the Health Services

Research Administration in the US Department of Health and Human Services, and the Department of Defense. Outside the United States, excellent research is conducted in Australia and Europe.

As of 2006, only a few health insurers in the United States will reimburse for telerehabilitation services. If the research shows that tele-assessments and tele-therapy are equivalent to clinical encounters, it is more likely that insurers and Medicare will cover telerehabilitation services.

Technologies

Plain old telephone service (POTS) with videophones/phones in telerehabilitation:

- There are several types of connections used with real time exchanges. Plain old telephone service (POTS) uses standard analog telephone lines. Videophones are used with POTS lines and include a camera, display screen, and telephone. Videophones use telephone lines that are available in most homes, so are easy to set up; however small display screens make them problematic for individuals with vision problems. This can be solved by using a large screen or television as a screen.

Videotelephony/Videotelephony in telerehabilitation:

- The use of improved quality video-assisted telecommunication devices, such as videoconferencing, webcams and telepresence to assist in treatments.

Virtual reality/Virtual reality in telerehabilitation:

- Virtual reality in telerehabilitation is one of the newest tools available in that area. This computer technology allows the development of three-dimensional virtual environments.

- Motion technology/Motion technology in telerehabilitation.

- Web-based approaches/Web-based approaches in telerehabilitation.

- Applications that run over the internet, just as if they were installed in your computer (called Rich Internet Applications), represent a new direction in software development. A person subscribes to the website rather than purchase the software. Any updates or changes to the software system are instantly available to all subscribers. The applications can be accessed from any location where one has access to an internet connected computer. Likewise, a patient's data is accessible from where ever the therapist is located. Neither the application nor the patient's data is tied to one computer.

- Sensors and body monitoring/Sensors and body monitoring in telerehabilitation.

- Haptic technology/Haptic technology in telerehabilitation.
- Artificial intelligence/Artificial intelligence in telerehabilitation.
- Wireless technology/Wireless technology in telerehabilitation.
- PDAs/PDA in telerehabilitation.
- Mobile telephony/Mobile telephony in telerehabilitation.
- Electronic medical records/Electronic medical record telerehabilitation.
- Mobile apps/Mobile apps telerehabilitation.

Clinical Applications

Speech-language Pathology

The clinical services provided by speech-language pathology readily lend themselves to telerehabilitation applications due to the emphasis on auditory and visual communicative interaction between the client and the clinician. As a result, the number of telerehabilitation applications in speech-language pathology tend to outnumber those in other allied health professions. To date, applications have been developed to assess and/or treat acquired adult speech and language disorders, stuttering, voice disorders, speech disorders in children, and swallowing dysfunction. The technology involved in these applications has ranged from the simple telephone (Plain Old Telephone System – POTS) to the use of dedicated Internet-based videoconferencing systems.

Early applications to assess and treat acquired adult speech and language disorders involved the use of the telephone to treat patients with aphasia and motor speech disorders, a computer controlled video laserdisc over the telephone and a closed-circuit television system to assess speech and language disorders, and a satellite-based videoconferencing system to assess patients in rural areas. More recent applications have involved the use of sophisticated Internet-based videoconferencing systems with dedicated software which enable the assessment of language disorders, the treatment of language disorders and the assessment and treatment of motor speech disorders following brain impairment and Parkinson's disease. Collectively, these studies have revealed positive treatment outcomes, while assessment and diagnoses have been found to be comparable to face-to-face evaluations.

The treatment of stuttering has been adapted to a telerehabilitation environment with notable success. Two Australian studies involving the distance delivery of the Lidcombe program to children who stutter have utilized the telephone in conjunction with offline video recordings to successfully treat several children. Overall, the parents and children responded positively to the program delivered at a distant. Using a high speed videoconferencing system link, Sicotte, Lehoux, Fortier-Blanc and Leblanc assessed and treated six children and adolescents with a positive reduction in the frequency of dysfluency that was maintained six months later. In addition, a videoconferencing platform has been used successfully to provide follow-up treatment to an adult who had previously received intensive therapy.

Reports of telerehabilitation applications in paediatric speech and language disorders are sparse. A recent Australian pilot study has investigated the feasibility of an Internet-based assessment of speech disorder in six children. High levels of agreement between the online and face-to-face clinicians for single-word articulation, speech intelligibility, and oro-motor tasks were obtained suggesting that the Internet-based protocol had the potential to be a reliable method for assessing paediatric speech disorders.

Voice therapy across a variety of types of voice disorders has been shown to be effectively delivered via a telerehabilitation application. Mashima using PC based videoconferencing and speech analysis software compared 23 patients treated online with 28 persons treated face-to-face. The authors reported positive post treatment results with no significant difference in measures between the traditional and videoconferencing group, suggesting that the majority of traditional voice therapy techniques can be applied to distance treatment.

Although obvious limitations exist, telerehabilitation applications for the assessment of swallowing function have also been used with success. Lalor, Brown and Cranfield were able to obtain an initial assessment of the nature and extent of swallowing dysfunction in an adult via a videoconferencing link although a more complete evaluation was restricted due to the inability to physically determine the degree of laryngeal movement. A more sophisticated telerehabilitation application for the assessment of swallowing was developed by Perlman and Witthawaskul who described the use of real-time videofluoroscopic examination via the Internet. This system enabled the capture and display of images in real-time with only a three to five second delay.There has been considerable research into the assessment and treatment of dysphagia via telerehabilitation, including cost analyses, leading to the establishment of sustainable telerehabilitation services.

There continues to be a need for ongoing research to develop and validate the use of telerehabilitation applications in speech-language pathology in a greater number and variety of adult and paediatric communication and swallowing disorders.

Disciplines and Therapies

- Speech-language pathology.
- Audiology.
- Physical therapy.

- Occupational therapy.
- Psychology.
- Nursing.
- Social work.
- Rehabilitation counseling/Vocational rehabilitation.

Medicine Ball

A medicine ball (also known as an exercise ball, a med ball, or a fitness ball) is a weighted ball roughly the diameter of the shoulders (approx. 13.7 inches), often used for rehabilitation and strength training. The medicine ball also serves an important role in the field of sports medicine to improve strength and neuromuscular coordination. It is distinct from the inflated exercise ball, which is larger (up to 36″ diameter).

Medicine balls are usually sold as 2–25 lb (1–11 kg) balls and are used effectively in ballistic training to increase explosive power in athletes in all sports, e.g. throwing the medicine ball or jumping whilst holding it. Some medicine balls are up to 14″ (approx. 36 cm) in diameter and up to 14 lbs weight, or in the form of weighted basketballs.

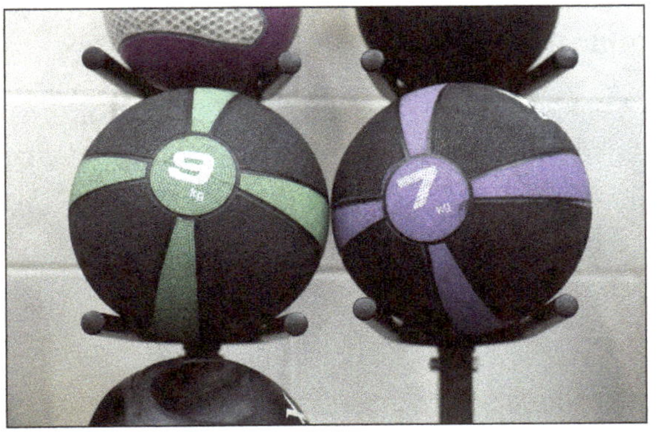

Medicine ball training is one of the oldest forms of strength and conditioning used to improve health, explosive power, and speed. Several styles and sizes exist – some are made of rubber or leather, some absorb load and others bounce really high.

Medicine ball training is suitable for all ages, fitness levels and sizes. There are many advantages to training with medicine balls. They allow for improved range of motion, core strength, coordination, flexibility, joint integrity, and upper and lower body strength.

Medicine balls are ideal for building explosive strength that's so important for sports performance. The freedom of movement allows for endless variations of exercises that can be tailored to your needs and more importantly, it teaches the body to work as an integrated system, which is key for improving athleticism and sport performance.

Core Benefits

Improving core strength, movement and stability – abdominals, lower back, hips and spine. The core is the body's centre of power. Using a medicine ball to train the core is perfect because you can perform so many functional movements similar to those that you do in everyday life. Instead of isolating certain muscle groups, you are able to train many different core muscles at once with the medicine ball.

Upper and Lower Strength

At the same time you're improving your core strength and stability, you're also developing upper and lower body strength. A medicine ball strengthen your legs and core when you do squats and lunges. You can develop explosive strength in you upper body by throwing the ball hard against the ground repeatedly with as much force as you can. Also it improves your balance.

Re-gaining Strength

Another great way to use medicine ball training is for rehab, but make sure you check with your doctor or therapist before doing so. Holding a medicine ball instead of dumbbells or a kettle bell adds an element of variety and fun to a workout. The exercises you can do with them are almost limitless.

Medicine balls come in a variety of weights. Start with a light one, especially if you've never worked with one before. You can always use a heavier one as your fitness level increases.

Diathermy

Diathermy is electrically induced heat or the use of high-frequency electromagnetic currents as a form of physical therapy and in surgical procedures. The earliest observations on the reactions of high-frequency electromagnetic currents upon the human organism were made by Jacques Arsene d'Arsonval. The field was pioneered in 1907 by German physician Karl Franz Nagelschmidt, who coined the term.

Diathermy is commonly used for muscle relaxation, and to induce deep heating in tissue for therapeutic purposes in medicine. It is used in physical therapy to deliver moderate heat directly to pathologic lesions in the deeper tissues of the body.

Diathermy is produced by three techniques: ultrasound (*ultrasonic diathermy*), shortwave radio frequencies in the range 1–100 MHz (*shortwave diathermy*) or microwaves typically in the 915 MHz or 2.45 GHz bands (*microwave diathermy*), the methods differing mainly in their penetration capability. It exerts physical effects and elicits a spectrum of physiological responses.

The same techniques are also used to create higher tissue temperatures to destroy neoplasms (cancer and tumors), warts, and infected tissues; this is called hyperthermia treatment. In surgery diathermy is used to cauterize blood vessels to prevent excessive bleeding. The technique is particularly valuable in neurosurgery and surgery of the eye.

Uses

Physical Therapy

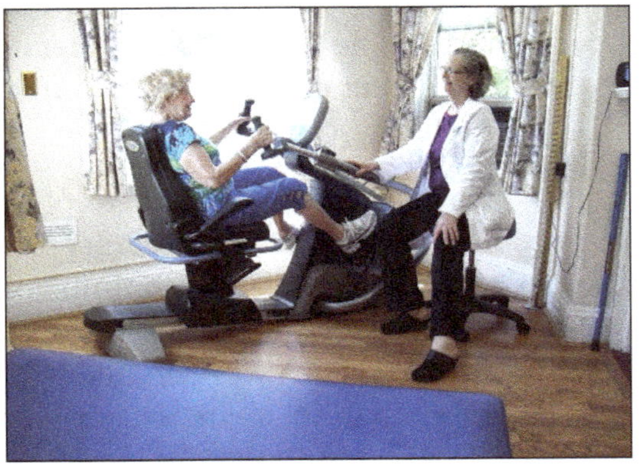

The three forms of diathermy employed by physical therapists are ultrasound, short wave and microwave. The application of moderate heat by diathermy increases blood flow and speeds up metabolism and the rate of ion diffusion across cellular membranes. The fibrous tissues in tendons, joint capsules, and scars are more easily stretched when subjected to heat, thus facilitating the relief of stiffness of joints and promoting relaxation of the muscles and decrease of muscle spasms.

Ultrasound

Ultrasound diathermy employs high-frequency acoustic vibrations which, when propelled through the tissues, are converted into heat. This type of diathermy is especially useful in the delivery of heat to selected musculatures and structures because there is a difference in the sensitivity of various fibers to the acoustic vibrations; some are more absorptive and some are more reflective. For example, in subcutaneous fat, relatively little energy is converted into heat, but in muscle tissues there is a much higher rate of conversion to heat.

The therapeutic ultrasound apparatus generates a high-frequency alternating current, which is then converted into acoustic vibrations. The apparatus is moved slowly across the surface of the part being treated. Ultrasound is a very effective agent for the application of heat, but it should be used only by a therapist who is fully aware of its potential hazards and the contraindications for its use.

Short Wave

Short wave diathermy machines use two condenser plates that are placed on either side of the body part to be treated. Another mode of application is by induction coils that are pliable and can be molded to fit the part of the body under treatment. As the high-frequency waves travel through the body tissues between the condensers or the coils, they are converted into heat. The degree of heat and depth of penetration depend in part on the absorptive and resistance properties of the tissues that the waves encounter.

Short wave diathermy operations use the ISM band frequencies of 13.56, 27.12, and 40.68 megahertz. Most commercial machines operate at a frequency of 27.12 MHz, a wavelength of approximately 11 meters.

Short wave diathermy usually is prescribed for treatment of deep muscles and joints that are covered with a heavy soft-tissue mass, for example, the hip. In some instances short wave diathermy may be applied to localize deep inflammatory processes, as in pelvic inflammatory disease. Short wave diathermy can also be used for hyperthermia therapy, as an adjuvant to radiation in cancer treatment. Typically, hyperthermia would be added twice a week before radiation, as shown in the photograph from a 2010 clinical trial at Mahavir Cancer Sansthan in Patna, India.

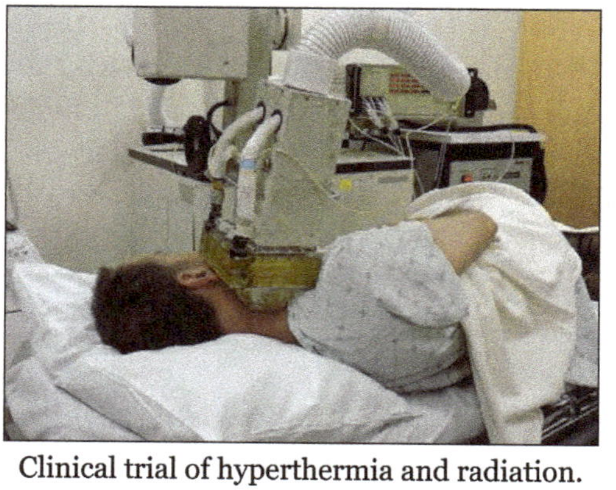

Clinical trial of hyperthermia and radiation.

Microwave

Microwave diathermy uses microwaves, radio waves which are higher in frequency and shorter in wavelength than the short waves above. Microwaves, which are also used in radar, have a frequency above 300 MHz and a wavelength less than one meter. Most, if not all, of the therapeutic effects of microwave therapy are related to the conversion of energy into heat and its distribution throughout the body tissues. This mode of diathermy is considered to be the easiest to use, but the microwaves have a relatively poor depth of penetration.

Microwaves cannot be used in high dosage on edematous tissue, over wet dressings, or near metallic implants in the body because of the danger of local burns. Microwaves and short waves cannot be used on or near persons with implanted electronic cardiac pacemakers.

Hyperthermia induced by microwave diathermy raises the temperature of deep tissues from 41 °C to 45 °C using electromagnetic power. The biological mechanism that regulates the relationship between the thermal dose and the healing process of soft tissues with low or high water content or with low or high blood perfusion is still under study. Microwave diathermy treatment at 434 and 915 MHz can be effective in the short-term management of musculo-skeletal injuries.

Hyperthermia is safe if the temperature is kept under 45 °C or 113 °F. The absolute temperature is, however, not sufficient to predict the damage that it may produce.

Microwave diathermy-induced hyperthermia produced short-term pain relief in established supraspinatus tendinopathy.

The physical characteristics of most of the devices used clinically to heat tissues have been proved to be inefficient to reach the necessary therapeutic heating patterns in the range of depth of the damage tissue. The preliminary studies performed with new microwave devices working at 434 MHz have demonstrated encouraging results. Nevertheless, adequately designed prospective-controlled clinical studies need to be completed to confirm the therapeutic effectiveness of hyperthermia with large number of patients, longer-term follow-up and mixed populations.

Microwave diathermy is used in the management of superficial tumours with conventional radiotherapy and chemotherapy. Hyperthermia has been used in oncology for more than 35 years, in addition to radiotherapy, in the management of different tumours. In 1994, hyperthermia was introduced in several countries of the European Union as a modality for use in physical medicine and sports traumatology. Its use has been successfully extended to physical medicine and sports traumatology in Central and Southern Europe.

Surgery

Surgical diathermy is usually better known as "electrosurgery". Electrosurgery and surgical diathermy involve the use of high-frequency A.C. electric current in surgery as either a cutting modality, or else to cauterize small blood vessels to stop bleeding. This technique induces localized tissue burning and damage, the zone of which is controlled by the frequency and power of the device.

Some sources insist that electrosurgery be applied to surgery accomplished by high-frequency alternating current (AC) cutting, and that "electrocautery" be used only for the practice of cauterization with heated nichrome wires powered by direct current (DC), as in the handheld battery-operated portable cautery tools.

Types

Diathermy used in surgery is of typically two types:

- Monopolar, where electric current passes from one electrode near the tissue to be treated to other fixed electrode (indifferent electrode) elsewhere in the body. Usually this type of electrode is placed in contact with buttocks or around the leg.
- Bipolar, where both electrodes are mounted on same pen-like device and electric current passes only through the tissue being treated. Advantage of bipolar electrosurgery is that it prevents the flow of current through other tissues of the body and focuses only on the tissue in contact. This is useful in microsurgery and in patients with cardiac pacemaker.

Diathermy Risks

Burns from electrocautery generally arise from a faulty grounding pad or from an outbreak of a fire. Monopolar electrocautery works because radio frequency energy is concentrated by the surgical instrument's small surface area. The electrical circuit is completed by passing current through the patient's body to a conductive pad that is connected to the radio frequency generator. Because the pad's surface area is large relative to the instrument's tip, energy density across the pad is reliably low enough that no tissue injury occurs at the pad site. Electrical shocks and burns are possible, however, if the circuit is interrupted or energy is concentrated in some way. This can happen if the pad surface in contact is small, e.g. if the pad's electrolytic gel is dry, if the pad becomes disconnected from the radio frequency generator, or via a metal implant. Modern electrocautery systems are equipped with sensors to detect high resistance in the circuit that can prevent some injuries.

As with all forms of heat applications, care must be taken to avoid burns during diathermy treatments, especially in patients with decreased sensitivity to heat and cold. With electrocautery there have been reported cases of flash fires in the operating theatre related to heat generation meeting chemical flash points, especially in the presence of increased oxygen concentrations associated with anaesthetic.

Concerns have also been raised regarding the toxicity of surgical smoke produced by electrocautery. This has been shown to contain chemicals which may cause harm to patients, surgeons and/or operating theatre staff.

For patients that have a surgically implanted Spinal Cord Stimulator (SCS) system, diathermy can cause tissue damage through energy that is transferred into the implanted SCS components resulting in severe injury or death

Electrotherapy

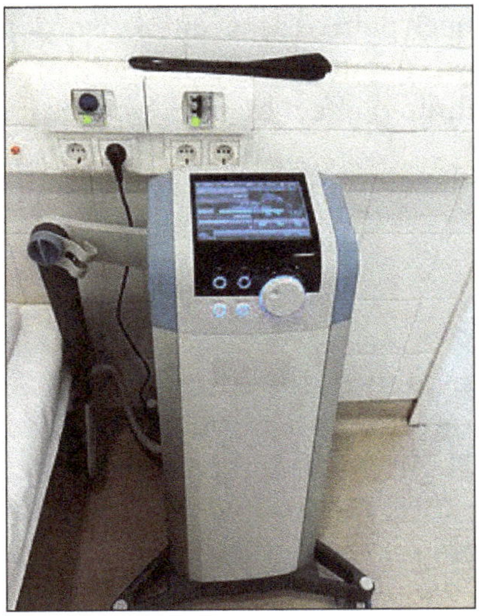

SIS electromagnetic therapy.

Electrotherapy is the use of electrical energy as a medical treatment. In medicine, the term *electrotherapy* can apply to a variety of treatments, including the use of electrical devices such as deep brain stimulators for neurological disease. The term has also been applied specifically to the use of electric current to speed wound healing. Additionally, the term "electrotherapy" or "electromagnetic therapy" has also been applied to a range of alternative medical devices and treatments.

Medical Uses

Electrotherapy is primarily used in physical therapy for relaxation of muscle spasms, prevention and retardation of disuse atrophy, increase of local blood circulation, muscle rehabilitation and re-education electrical muscle stimulation, maintaining and increasing range of motion, management of chronic and intractable pain, post-traumatic acute pain, post-surgical acute pain, immediate post-surgical stimulation of muscles to prevent venous thrombosis, wound healing and drug delivery.

Some of the treatment effectiveness mechanisms are little understood, with effectiveness and best practices for their use still anecdotal.

Musculoskeletal Conditions

In general, there is little evidence that electrotherapy is effective in the management of musculoskeletal conditions. In particular, there is no evidence that electrotherapy is effective in the relief of pain arising from osteoarthritis, and little to no evidence available to support electrotherapy for the management of fibromyalgia.

Neck and Back Pain

A review found that, "in evidence of no effectiveness," clinicians should not offer electrotherapy for the treatment of neck pain or associated disorders. Earlier reviews found that no conclusions could be drawn about the effectiveness of electrotherapy for neck pain, and that electrotherapy has limited effect on neck pain as measured by clinical results.

A review found that the evidence for electrotherapy in pregnancy-related lower back pain is "very limited".

Shoulder Disorders

A review found insufficient evidence to determine whether electrotherapy was better than exercise at treating adhesive capsulitis. As of 2004, there is insufficient evidence to draw conclusions about any intervention for rotator cuff pathology, including electrotherapy; furthermore, methodological problems precluded drawing conclusions about the efficacy of *any* rehabilitation method for impingement syndrome.

Other Musculoskeletal Disorders

There is limited, low quality evidence for a slight benefit of noxious-level electrotherapy in the treatment of epicondylitis.

A review found that "Small, single studies showed that some electrotherapy modalities may be beneficial" in rehabilitating ankle bone fractures. However, a review found it to be ineffective in healing long-bone fractures.

A review found that evidence that electrotherapy contributes to recovery from knee conditions is of "limited quality".

Chronic Pain

A review found "weaker evidence" that pulsating electromagnetic fields could be effective in treating recurrent headaches. A review found that supporting evidence for electrotherapy as a treatment for complex regional pain syndrome is "absent or unclear."

Gait Training

Gait training or gait rehabilitation is the act of learning how to walk, either as a child, or, more frequently, after sustaining an injury or disability. The process of relearning how to walk is generally facilitated by physical therapists, or physiotherapists. The most common cause for gait impairment is due to an injury of one or both legs. Gait training is not simply re-educating a patient on how to walk, but also includes an initial assessment of their gait cycle, creation of a plan to address the problem, as well as teaching the patient on how to walk on different surfaces. Assistive devices are often used in gait training, especially with those who have had surgery or an injury on their legs, but also with those who have balance or strength impairments as well. Gait training can be useful for people with the following conditions:

- Amputation.
- Osteoarthritis.
- Muscular dystrophy.
- Cerebral palsy.
- Stroke.
- Parkinson's disease.
- Multiple sclerosis.
- Brain and spinal cord injuries.
- After surgery.
- Sports injury.

Although gait training with parallel bars, treadmills and support systems can be beneficial, the long-term aim of gait training is usually to reduce patients' dependence on such technology in order to walk more in their daily lives.

Gait Cycle

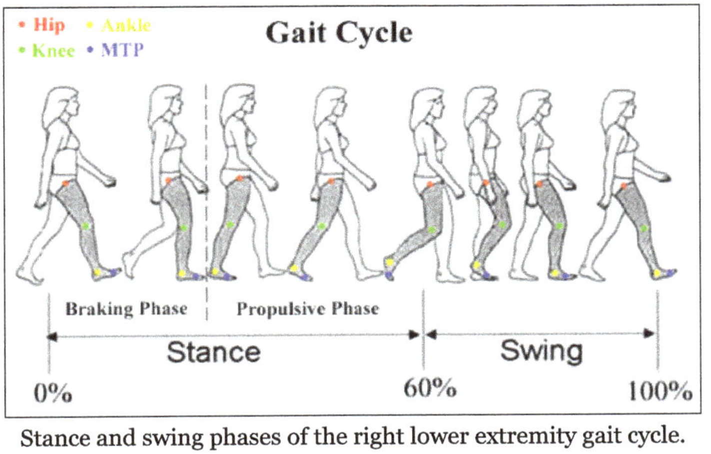

Stance and swing phases of the right lower extremity gait cycle.

A gait cycle is defined as the progression of movements that occurs before one leg can return to a certain position during walking, or ambulation. One example of a full gait cycle is the period it takes for a foot to leave the ground until the same leaves the ground again. An understanding of a normal gait cycle and how it progresses is crucial to determining how much assistance a patient needs in order to return to functional ambulation. How long the gait cycle lasts depends on multiple factors, such as age, walking surface, and walking speed.

There are two main phases to the gait cycle.

Stance

The stance phase begins when the foot first makes contact with the ground (initial contact), and the weight of the body is borne by that limb. This phase is approximately 60% of the gait cycle and takes about 0.6 seconds to complete at a normal walking speed. Included in the stance phase are another four intervals, which are: load response, midstance, terminal stance, and preswing. Load response occurs when the body weight is borne by the single foot while the other foot begins to lift off the ground to start its swing phase. At midstance the body is supported fully by one leg and the other is no longer in contact with the ground. During terminal stance body weight is still supported on one leg, however the heel of that leg is beginning to lift off, and the center of gravity is in front of the foot still in contact with the ground. Finally at preswing the toe of the stance foot comes off the ground, and the weight is now transferred to the leg that was previously in the swing phase.

Swing

The swing phase occurs when the foot is not in contact with the ground, and constitutes about 40% of the gait cycle. There are three intervals to this phase: initial swing, midswing, and terminal swing. During initial swing, the foot is lifted off the floor. Next it moves into midswing, when the lower leg is straight and is perpendicular to the floor. Finally, at the terminal phase, the foot comes back into contact with the floor again and restarts the cycle beginning in initial contact of the stance phase.

Assistive Devices

Assistive devices (ADs) are given to patients who have difficulty maintaining a regular gait cycle or balance due to an injury to one or both of their legs. Other factors that would necessitate use of an AD include loss of perception in the legs, weakness of the legs, pain while walking, and a history of falling, among other indications. Not only does an AD provide extra support, it can also protect the injured leg and prevent it from being further aggravated due to weight bearing requirements. Different ADs are assigned to each patient depending on the severity of their condition and how much extra support they need provided. The following list presents the ADs from the least supportive to the most supportive.

- Straight cane.
- Lofstrand crutches.

- Axillary crutches.
- Walker.
- Parallel Bar.

Weight Bearing Status

The type of gait that a patient is instructed in is based on their weight-bearing status, or how much of their body weight can be supported on their legs, coordination, and strength. There are different levels of weight-bearing status that is determined by the physician. The weight-bearing status of a patient generally changes as treatment progresses, but each progression needs to be approved by the physician. In many cases the easiest way to monitor a patient's weight bearing status is to use two scales, one under each foot, and to adjust the weight on each foot until the injured foot is supported the desired amount of weight.

There are four different weight-bearing statuses:

- Non-Weight Bearing (NWB).
- Touch-Down Weight Bearing (TDWB) or Toe Touch Weight Bearing (TTWB).
- Partial Weight Bearing (PWB).
- Weight Bearing as Tolerated (WBAT).

In NWB, the patient is not allowed to bear any weight on their injured leg. For TTWB, the amount of weight placed on the leg is defined in many ways, such as being approximately 20% of body weight, being 10 to 15 kg of weight, or being equal to or less than a weight that would crush eggshells. The portion of weight that is allowed to be borne on the injured leg in PWB is generally given as a percentage, such as 25% or 50%, however with a percentage the amount of weight that is supported changes as the person's weight changes as well. In WBAT the person is allowed to bear as much weight as pain allows, provided that the pain level does not become difficult to tolerate.

Gait Training using Assistive Devices

There are multiple possible gait patterns that can be taught to the patient, and the one that is taught depends on the patient's capability and coordination. Parallel bars may be used to help with gait training, especially in the early stages when a patient is first learning or re-learning to walk. They involve a person walking between two handrails to support themselves, often with the therapist either helping to support the patient or physically moving the patient's legs. A gait belt is also utilized by the physical therapist in order to support the patient and to prevent them from falling or placing too much weight on the injured leg.

Two-point Gait Pattern

The two-point gait pattern closely imitates a unaffected gait pattern, but includes the use of two crutches or two canes with one on either side of the body. In this pattern one crutch and the leg opposite to the crutch is moved in unison. For example if the right crutch is moved forward, then the left leg would advance with it. This gait pattern requires a high level of coordination and balance.

Another two-point gait pattern is the modified two-point pattern. In this pattern there is only use of one crutch or cane on the side opposite to the injured leg, therefore there can not be any weight bearing restriction but is more used to provide extra balance. For this pattern the AD is move simultaneously with the injured leg.

Three-point Gait Pattern

A three-point gait pattern can be used with patients who are NWB, however requires a much higher energy output and requires the patient to have good balance as well as strong upper limbs. A walker or two crutches must be used, as this pattern can not be performed with the use of a single cane. For this pattern the AD is advanced first, then the uninjured leg is moved up as the body is supported on the AD. The uninjured leg can either be brought up to be level with the AD (swing to) or brought up to be ahead of the AD (swing through).

There is also a modified three-point gait pattern which can be used with patients who are PWB on their injured leg but full weight bearing (FWB) on their uninjured leg. This pattern also requires the use of 2 crutches or a walker, but is slower and more stable than the three-point gait pattern. In the modified pattern, the AD is advanced first, followed by the injured leg that has a PWB status, then finally the uninjured leg is moved up. Just as in the three-point gait pattern the patient may use a swing to or a swing through pattern.

Stairs

Ascending Stairs

Two crutches or a cane can be used to ascending a flight of stairs. Although a walker may also be used, it is not recommended to be used to climb stairs longer than 2 or 3 steps. If the patient is using two crutches, then both crutches are held in one hand while the other hand grips the handrail. If there is no handrail or if it the two crutches can not be held in one hand, both crutches may be used without use of the handrail, although this method is not recommended for taking more than 2 or 3 steps. The order of events goes: uninjured foot, crutches or cane, injured foot. This process is repeated until the patient reaches the top of the stairs.

Descending Stairs

Just as in ascending stairs, two crutches or a cane may be used to descend a flight of stairs, and use of a walker is not recommended for climbing more than 2 or 3 steps. Both crutches should be used if the handrail is unstable or if the two crutches are not able to be held securely in one hand. The crutches or cane descends to the first step, then is followed by the injured leg, then finally the uninjured leg. This process is repeated until the bottom of the stairs is reached.

Heat Therapy

Heat therapy, also called thermotherapy, is the use of heat in therapy, such as for pain relief and health. It can take the form of a hot cloth, hot water bottle, ultrasound, heating pad, hydrocollator packs, whirlpool baths, cordless FIR heat therapy wraps, and others. It can be beneficial to those with arthritis and stiff muscles and injuries to the deep tissue of the skin. Heat may be an effective self-care treatment for conditions like rheumatoid arthritis.

Heat therapy is most commonly used for rehabilitation purposes. The therapeutic effects of heat include increasing the extensibility of collagen tissues; decreasing joint stiffness; reducing pain; relieving muscle spasms; reducing inflammation, edema, and aids in the post acute phase of healing; and increasing blood flow. The increased blood flow to the affected area provides proteins, nutrients, and oxygen for better healing.

Application

Direct Contact

Moist heat therapy has been believed to be more effective at warming tissues than dry heat, because water transfers heat more quickly than air. Clinical studies do not support the popular belief that moist heat is more effective than dry heat. Moist heat results in the perception that the tissue is heated more deeply. In fact, recent studies indicate that vasodilation, the expansion of the blood capillaries (vessels) to allow more blood flow, is improved with dry heat therapy. Expansion of the blood capillaries is the primary objective of heat therapy. Heat therapy increases the effect on muscles, joints, and soft tissue. Heat is typically applied by placing a warming device on the relevant body part.

Newer breeds of heat therapy devices combine a carbon fiber heater with a cordless rechargeable lithium battery and are built into the specific body wrap (*i.e.*, shoulder wrap or back wrap) for targeted heat therapy. Such devices can be used as alternatives to chemical or plugged-in heating pads, but have not been shown to improve the clinical benefit. All devices primarily provide heat to promote vasodilation.

Infrared Radiation

Infrared radiation is a convenient system to heat parts of our body. It has the advantage over direct contact in that radiation can heat directly the area where the blood capillaries and neuron terminals are. When heat comes from a direct contact source it has to heat the external layer of the skin, and heat is transferred to the deeper layer by conduction. Since heat conduction needs a temperature gradient to proceed, and there is a maximum temperature that can be safely used (around 42 °C), this means lower temperature where warming is needed.

Infrared (IR for short) is the part of the electromagnetic radiation spectrum comprised between 0.78 μm and 1 mm wavelength. It is usually divided into three segments:

- IR-A, from 0.78 to 1.4 μm.
- IR-B, from 1.4 to 3 μm.
- IR-C, from 3 μm to 1 mm.

IR radiation is more useful than the visible radiation for heating our body, because we absorb most of it, compared to a strong reflection of visible light. Penetration depth of infrared radiation in our skin is dependent of wavelength. IR-A is the most penetrating, and reaches some millimeters, IR-B penetrates into the dermis (about 1 mm), and IR-C is mostly absorbed in the external layer of the epidermis (stratum corneum). For this reason the infrared lamps used for therapeutic purposes produce mainly IR-A radiation.

Mechanism of Action and Indications

Heat creates higher tissue temperatures, which produces vasodilation that increases the supply of oxygen and nutrients and the elimination of carbon dioxide and metabolic waste. Heat therapy is useful for muscle spasms, myalgia, fibromyalgia, contracture, bursitis.

Moist heat can be used on abscesses to help drain the abscess faster. A study from 2005 showed heat therapy to be effective in treating leishmaniasis, a tropical parasitic skin infection.

Heat therapy is also sometimes used in cancer treatment to augment the effect of chemotherapy or radiotherapy, but it is not enough to kill cancer cells on its own.

Heat therapy is contraindicated in case of acute injury and bleeding disorders (because of vasodilation), tissues with a severe lack of sensitivity, scars and in tissues with inadequate vascular supply (because of increased metabolic rate and demand which a tissue with poor blood supply may fail to meet resulting in ischemia).

The use of Heat therapy for deep-seated tissue can be treated with shortwave, microwave, and ultrasonic waves. This produces a high temperature that penetrates deeper. Shortwave produces a 27MHz current, microwaves use 915 and 2456 MHz, and ultrasound is an acoustic vibration of 1MHz. The way ultrasonic waves work is they selectively superimpose the incoming wave and increase the energy for absorption, and the significant part of the longitudinal compression gets converted into shear waves. When they are rapidly absorbed, the interface between soft tissue and bone is selectively heated.

For Headaches

Heat therapy can be used for the treatment of headaches and migraines. Many people who suffer from chronic headaches also suffer from tight muscles in their neck and upper back. The application of constant heat to the back/upper back area can help to release the tension associated with headache pain. In order to achieve heat therapy for headaches, many use microwaveable pads which can often overheat, potentially leading to injury, and lose their heat after a few minutes. Some new products use heated water, running through pads, to maintain a constant temperature, allowing headache sufferers to use hands-free heat therapy in the treatment of their headache pain.

Therapeutic Benefits

Thermotherapy increase the extensibility of collagen tissues. Using heat, it can relieve the stiffness in joints in different cases. Shortwave and Microwave heat application may reduce muscle spasms, and selective heating with microwaves can accelerate absorption of hematomas. This will, in turn, allow the stiff muscle to stretch. Ultrasounds are not absorbed significantly in homogenous muscle. Heat therapy using hyperthermia has been used to treat cancer in combination with ionizing radiation.

Splint

A splint is defined as "a rigid or flexible device that maintains in position a displaced or movable part; also used to keep in place and protect an injured part" or as "a rigid or flexible material used to protect, immobilize, or restrict motion in a part." Splints can be used for injuries that are not severe enough to immobilize the entire injured structure of the body. For instance, a splint can be used for certain fractures, soft tissue sprains, tendon injuries, or injuries awaiting orthopedic treatment. A splint may be static, not allowing motion, or dynamic, allowing controlled motion. Splints can also be used to relieve pain in damaged joints. Splints are quick and easy to apply and do not require a plastering technique. Splints are often made out of some kind of flexible material and a firm pole-like structure for stability. They often buckle or Velcro together.

Uses

- By the emergency medical services or by volunteer first responders, to temporarily immobilize a fractured limb before transportation.

- By allied health professionals such as occupational therapists, physiotherapists and orthotists, to immobilize an articulation (e.g. the knee) that can be freed while not standing (e.g. during sleep).
- By athletic trainers to immobilize an injured bone or joint to facilitate safer transportation of the injured person.
- By emergency department (ED) physicians to stabilize fractures or sprains until follow-up appointment with an orthopedist.

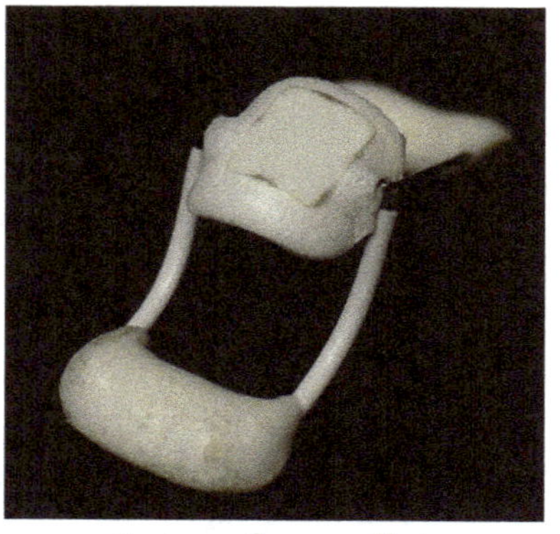

Capener finger splint.

Types

- Ankle stirrup – Used for the ankles.
- Finger splints – Used for the fingers. A "mallet" or baseball finger is a rupture of the extensor tendon and sometimes including a fracture. While surgery may be necessary such an injury may heal if placed in a finger splint.

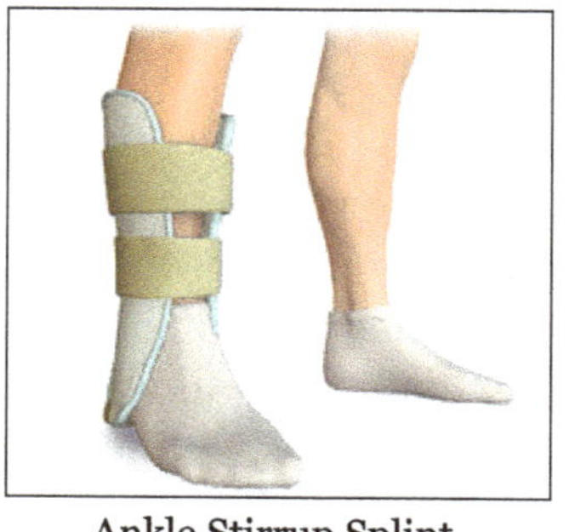

Ankle Stirrup Splint.

- Nasal splint.
- Posterior lower leg.
- Posterior full leg.
- Posterior elbow.

- Sugar tong – Used for the forearm or wrist. They are named "sugar-tong" due to their long, U-shaped characteristics, similar to a type of utensil used to pick up sugar cubes.
- Thumb spica – Used for the thumb.
- Ulnar gutter – Used for the forearm to the palm.
- Volar wrist splint – Used for the wrist.
- Wrist/arm splint – Used for the wrist or arm.

Traction

Traction refers to the set of mechanisms for straightening broken bones or relieving pressure on the spine and skeletal system. There are two types of traction: skin traction and skeletal traction. They are used in orthopedic medicine.

Techniques

Traction procedures are largely replaced now by more modern techniques, but certain approaches are still used today:

- Milwaukee brace.
- Bryant's traction.
- Buck's traction, involving skin traction. It is widely used for femoral fractures, low back pain, acetabular fractures and hip fractures. Skin traction rarely causes fracture reduction, but reduces pain and maintains the length of the bone.
- Dunlop's traction – humeral fractures in children.
- Russell's traction.

Skeletal Traction

Although the use of traction has decreased over the years, an increasing number of orthopaedic practitioners are using traction in conjunction with bracing.

Harrison found that mirror image (opposite posture) postural corrective exercises and a new method of lumbosacral tilt traction resulted in 50% reduction in trunk tilt and were associated with nearly resolved pain intensity in this patient population. These researchers felt that their findings warranted further study in the conservative treatment of chronic low back pain and spinal disorders.

Spinal Decompression

Spinal traction as a means of spinal decompression is often applied without directly touching bones as other methods of traction do. This is sometimes isolated inside-out by inflatable girdles or use of the transversus abdominis muscle. It is also done in conjunction with thigh-supported flexed-hip traction (inversion chairs, back hyperextensions) or done in conjunction with whole-leg traction (boots, tables) via inverted forms of suspension.

Traction of the spine (except the cervical) also occurs with upright suspension of the body from the arms, such as with pull-ups, dips, captain's chair, chinnings (chin up exercise) or other fitness movements with the feet dangling.

Purpose

The purpose of traction is to:

- Regain normal length and alignment of involved bone.
- Lessen or eliminate muscle spasms.
- Relieve pressure on nerves, especially spinal nerves.
- Prevent or reduce skeletal deformities or muscle contractures.
- To provide a fusiform tamponade around a bleeding vessel.

In most cases traction is only one part of the treatment plan of a patient needing such therapy. The physician's order will contain:

- Type of traction.
- Amount of weight to be applied.
- Frequency of neurovascular checks if more frequent than every four hours.
- Site care of inserted pins, wires, or tongs.
- The site and care of straps, harnesses and halters.
- The inclusion of any other physical restraints/straps or appliances (e.g., mouth guard).
- The discontinuation of traction.

Soft Tissue Therapy

Soft Tissue Therapy (STT) is the assessment, treatment and management of soft tissue injury, pain, and dysfunction of the musculoskeletal system.

A soft tissue therapist will use deep tissue massage skills to treat you along with manual stretching, myofascial release and trigger point therapy.

The soft tissues of the body refer to muscles, tendons, ligaments and fascia. Therapy of these soft tissues requires management, manipulation and rehabilitation to any individual regardless of whether they are involved in sport or not.

Patients will benefit from safe, effective and efficient results following treatment with a soft tissue therapist. The session differs to a general sports massage in a number of ways, firstly, clients are not all from a sport background, we treat everyone. Secondly, in your soft tissue therapy session a variety of other techniques may be used by the therapist to provide an appropriate treatment. These techniques include: muscle energy techniques, soft tissue release, assisted stretching, Deep Tissue Friction, Myofascial Release, Trigger Point Therapy, cupping and Acupuncture.

Sports Massage

Massage affects the soft tissues, but during treatment we often need to target the joints in tandem with soft tissue therapy. A brief overview of some principles behind joint techniques is given below:

Accessory Movements

The movements of a joint are of two types, physiological and accessory. Physiological movements are those which the athlete can perform actively, for example flexion and extension of the knee. Accessory movements cannot be produced actively as individual movements, but occur automatically between articulating surfaces of a joint as it moves. Three accessory movements are of particular importance when treating sports injuries: these are roll, slide and spin.

- Roll occurs when points at certain intervals on a moving surface contact points at the same intervals on the opposing surface. This is similar to a car tyre rolling over the road.
- Slide is seen if one point on the moving surface stays in contact with a variety of points on the opposing surface.
- Spin is a pure rotation around a mechanical axis. Usually when a joint moves, both slide and roll must take place. If roll alone were the only movement, the joint would sublux before any appreciable range had been achieved. If only slide occurred, the edges of the concave aspect of the joint would impinge on the opposing convex lip.

Close and Loose Pack

The two opposing surfaces of a joint do not fit together exactly; they are said to be non-congruent. But, with the joint in one particular position its surfaces will come as close together as they are able, and this is known as 'close pack'. In this position the joint capsule and ligaments twist and pull the joint surfaces together into approximation. The joint space is at a minimum and the concave surface of one bone fits tightly into the convex shape of the other. No further movement is possible in a joint which is close packed, and so this position is avoided when trying to mobilize the joint.

Loose pack position is exactly the opposite. As the joint surfaces are released from their close pack position, elastic recoil of the soft tissues surrounding the joint enables its surfaces to move apart, maximizing the joint space. The loose pack position is the resting position often taken up after injury because more joint fluid can accumulate. In loose pack positions joint play is possible. This consists of small accessory movements which give the joint its 'spring'. These are essential to the normal functioning of the joint and play a part in joint nutrition and combined movements.

Interestingly many fractures of the upper limb occur with a fall onto the outstretched arm, which is a close packed position, and many ligament sprains occur in loose packed position.

Table: Close packed and loose packed positions of selected joints.

Joint(s)	Close packed position	Loose packed (resting) position
Facet (spine)	Extension	Midway between flexion and extension
Temporomandibular	Clenched teeth	Mouth slightly open
Glenohumeral	Abduction and external rotation	55° abduction, 30° horizontal abduction, rotated so that the forearm is in the transverse plane
Acromioclavicular	Arm abduction to 30°	Arm resting by side, shoulder girdle in the physiological position
Sternoclavicular	Maximum shoulder elevation	Arm resting by side, shoulder girdle in the physiological position
Ulnohumeral (elbow)	Extension	70° elbow flexion, 10° forearm supination
Radiohumeral	Elbow flexed 90°, forearm supinated 5°	Full extension, full supination
Proximal radioulnar	5° supination	70° elbow flexion, 35° forearm supination
Distal radioulnar	5° supination	10° forearm supination
Radiocarpal (wrist)	Extension with ulnar deviation	Midway between flexion–extension (so that a straight line passes through the radius and third metacarpal) with slight ulnar deviation
First carpometacarpal	Full opposition	Midway between abduction-adduction and flexion-extension
Metacarpophalangeal (fingers)	Full flexion	Slight flexion
Metacarpophalangeal (thumb)	Full opposition	
Interphalangeal	Full extension	Slight flexion

Hip	Full extension, internal rotation and abduction	30° flexion, 30° abduction, and slight external rotation
Knee	Full extension and external rotation of the tibia	25° flexion
Talocrural (ankle)	Maximum dorsiflexion	10° plantarflexion, midway between maximum inversion and eversion
Subtalar	Full supination	Midway between extremes of inversion and eversion
Midtarsal	Full supination	Midway between extremes of range of movement
Tarsometatarsal	Full supination	Midway between extremes of range of movement
Metatarsophalangeal	Full extension	Neutral
Interphalangeal	Full extension	Slight flexion

Concept of Mobilization and Manipulation

Mobilization using Accessory Movements

Where pain and stiffness limit the normal (physiological) movement of a joint, rather than pressing further into this painful range, *accessory movements* may be used. By increasing the range available to accessory motion, the physiological range may also increase.

If pain is the dominant factor, this is treated first. When stiffness overshadows pain the aim is to increase the patient's range of motion even though some soreness may be produced during and following treatment. Most patients will present with a combination of pain and stiffness, and when there is doubt as to which is the predominant feature, pain is treated first.

When joint movement is limited, the point of limitation falls short of the anatomical range (that which is available to a joint because of its structure). As the joint is mobilized the point of limitation moves closer to the anatomical range. Within a range of movement four grades of mobilization techniques are used.

Grades of mobilization procedures:

- Grade I: Small amplitude movement near the starting position of the range.
- Grade II: Large amplitude movement occupying any free part of the range.
- Grade III: Large amplitude movement moving into stiffness.
- Grade IV: Small amplitude movement at the end of range.

Represented diagrammatically grades I and II do not reach the end range, and are used when pain is the predominant feature. Grades III and IV are performed to end-range movement and are used when stiffness is the main problem.

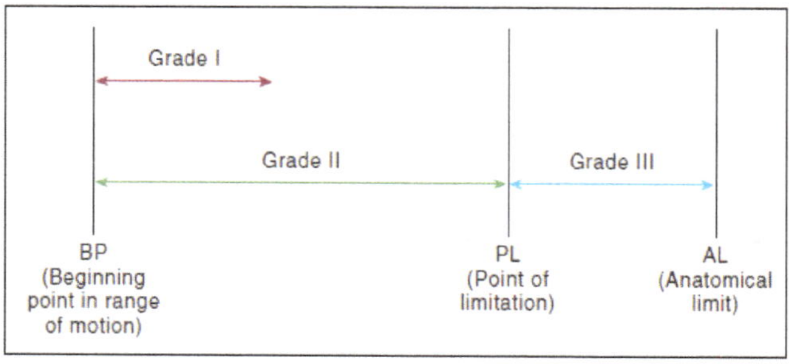

Grades of joint mobilization. A, starting point of movement range. B, anatomical limitation of range. L, limitation point due to pain.

A number of techniques may be used. In the knee, for example, lateral movements and anteroposterior (AP) movements are useful accessory movements for treatment, while normal bending and straightening (flexion and extension) represent the physiological movements which would be expected to increase as a result of joint mobilization.

References

- Manual-Therapy: physio-pedia.com, Retrieved 28 February, 2020
- Becker, BE and Cole, AJ (eds). 2011. Comprehensive aquatic therapy, 3rd edition. Washington State University Press. ISBN 978-0615365671
- What-is-soft-tissue-therapy: puresportsmed.com, Retrieved 13 July, 2020
- Fryer GA, Mudge JM, McLaughlin PA (2002). "The effect of talocrural joint manipulation on range of motion at the ankle" (PDF). Journal of Manipulative and Physiological Therapeutics. 25 (6): 384–90. doi:10.1067/mmt.2002.126129. PMID 12183696
- Benefits-using-medicine-ball: mywaffl.com, Retrieved 1 August, 2020
- Soft-tissue-therapy, medicine-and-dentistry: sciencedirect.com, Retrieved 19 May, 2020
- Mac Auley, D. C. (July 2001). "Ice therapy: how good is the evidence?". International Journal of Sports Medicine. 22 (5): 379–84. doi:10.1055/s-2001-15656. ISSN 0172-4622. PMID 11510876

Rehabilitation Exercises 5

- Stretching Exercises
- Foam Roller Exercises
- Plyometric Exercises
- Wrist and Hand Exercises

Rehabilitation exercises help in restoring lost skills and regaining maximum self-sufficiency. Stretching exercises, foam roller exercises, plyometric exercises, etc. are a few rehabilitation exercises. This chapter has been carefully written to provide an extensive understanding of these rehabilitation exercises.

Stretching Exercises

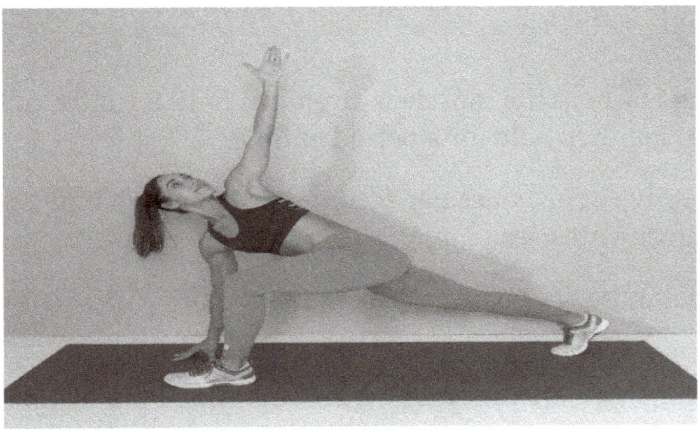

Stretching is a form of physical exercise in which a specific muscle or tendon (or muscle group) is deliberately flexed or stretched in order to improve the muscle's felt elasticity and achieve comfortable muscle tone. The result is a feeling of increased muscle control, flexibility, and range of motion. Stretching involves the performance of a controlled movement through the available ROM. It is good to use in advanced sports related rehabilitation and active sports persons.

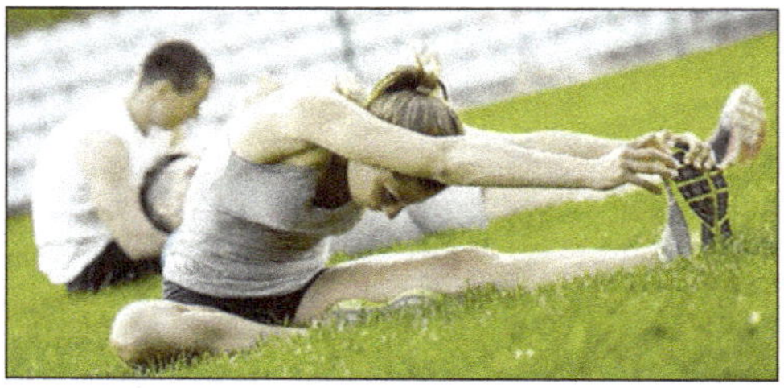

Benefits of Stretching

Flexibility is the range of movement at a joint. It means the same as mobility or suppleness and is important in sport. Stretching has a number of benefits including:

- Increasing range of motion.
- Preventing injury.
- Avoiding DOMS (delayed onset muscle soreness).
- Improving posture.
- Stress relief.
- Enhanced sports performance.

Types of Stretching

There are a number of different types of stretching exercises which can be done to improve flexibility. The most appropriate technique will depend on your specific aims and include:

- Static stretching is where the muscle is stretched until a gentle 'pull' or stretch on the muscle is felt then held for a period of time.
- PNF (proprioceptive neuromuscular facilitation) type techniques involve contracting and relaxing muscles.
- Dynamic stretching is very much in fashion these days, particularly in sport for warming up.
- Ballistic stretching is where the end range of movement of the joint is forced.
- Neural stretching refers to stretching the structures of the nervous system, for example, sciatic nerve stretches.

Foot and Ankle Stretching Exercises

Stretching exercises for the foot, ankle & shin, including the calf muscles (gastrocnemius and soleus), Tibialis Anterior, Extensor Digitorum Longus, Extensor Hallucis Longus, peroneal muscle, and plantar fascia. These stretches are important for recovering from lower leg injuries.

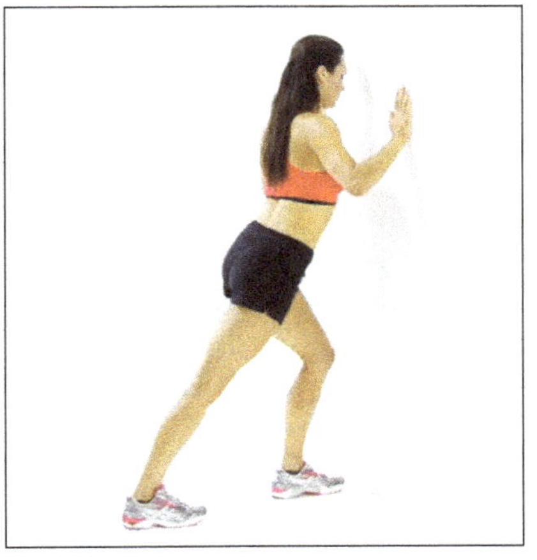

Thigh Stretching Exercises

Stretching exercises for the quadriceps and hamstring muscles are important for preventing and recovering from hamstring strains, thigh contusion, quadriceps strains, and groin injuries.

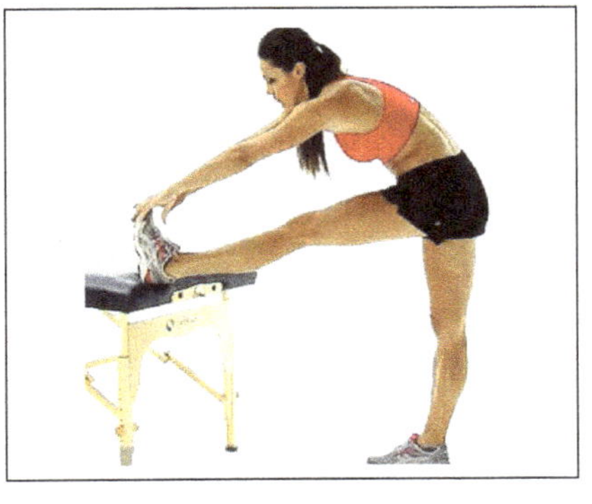

Hip and Groin Stretching Exercises

These exercises are important for recovering from groin strains, piriformis syndrome, and other hip and groin-related injuries.

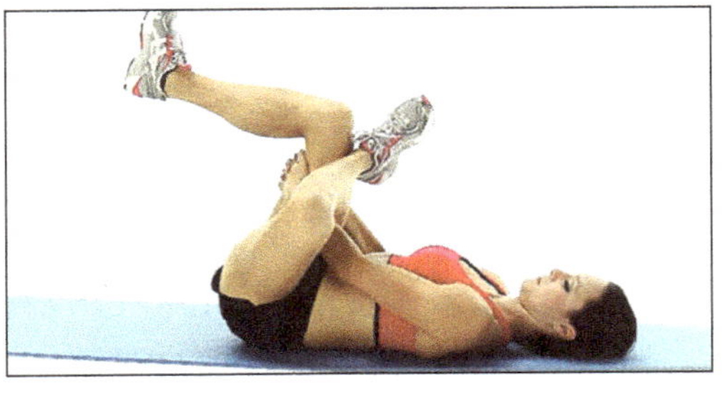

- Standing groin stretch.
- Long adductor stretch.
- Piriformis stretch.
- Hip flexor stretch.

Back Stretching Exercises

Back stretching is important to include in your general training routine to help prevent injury and even improve sports performance. If you have back pain or any kind of back injury then it is important to get professional advice as some back exercises may not be suitable.

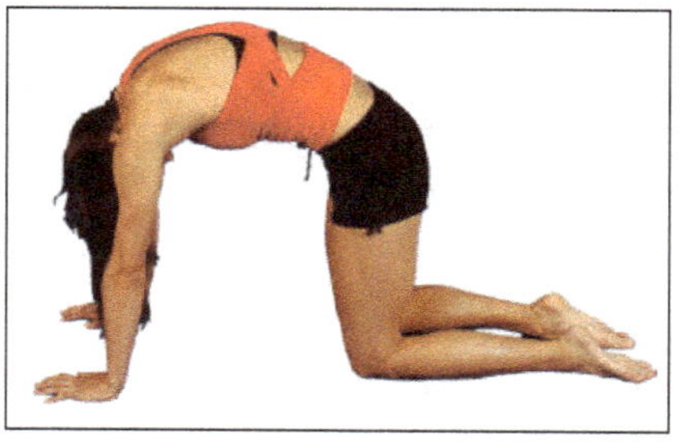

Shoulder Stretching Exercises

Shoulder stretching exercises, including anterior shoulder stretch, chest stretch, Triceps stretch, and Latissimus Dorsi stretch as well as partner-assisted exercises which can increase a range of motion still further in the shoulder joints.

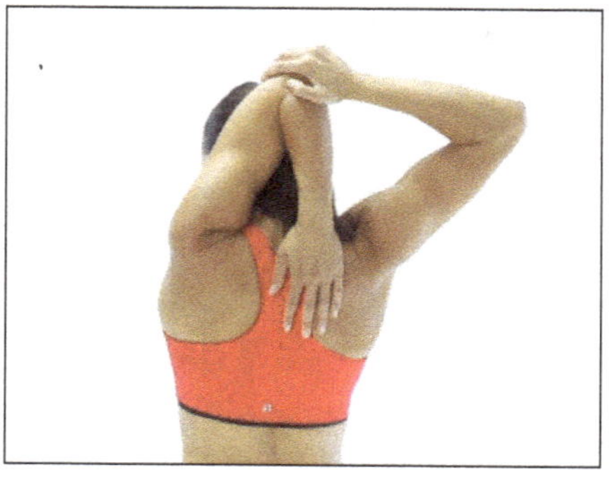

Elbow and Wrist Stretching

Elbow and arm stretching exercises are usually most important when rehabilitating an elbow or wrist injury, and include wrist flexors, wrist extensors, tennis elbow stretch, and triceps muscle. In particular, martial artists often do wrist and arm stretches as part of their warm-up.

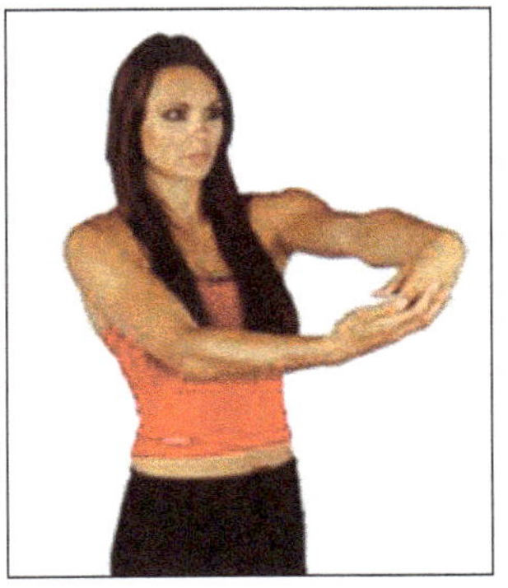

Neck Stretching Exercises

Stretching exercises for the neck including rotation stretch, forward and lateral flexion stretches, and Sternocleidomastoid stretch. Neck mobility exercises are also excellent for relieving the tension caused by too many hours sitting at a desk or in front of a computer.

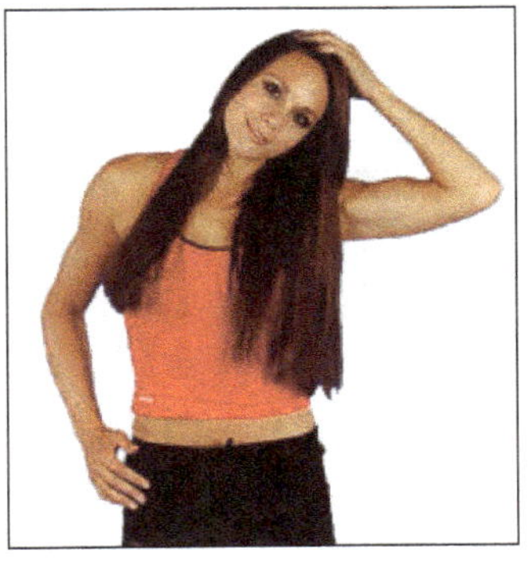

Foam Roller Exercises

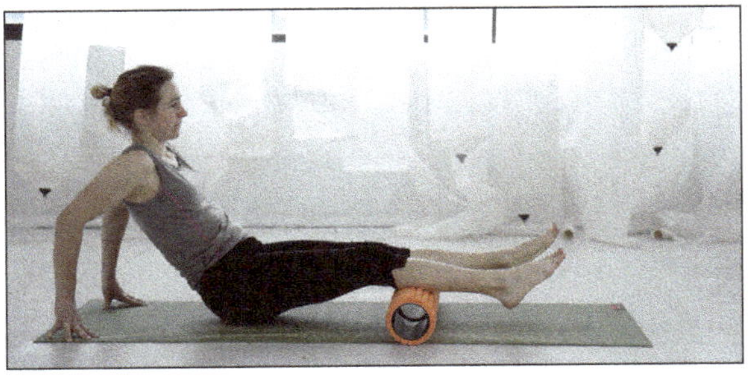

Foam rollers are a popular tool for helping athletes release muscle knots or trigger points. "Myofascial adhesions" is the physiological term for these inflexible areas that can be caused by muscle imbalance, overuse and injuries, among other things.

Many people develop a love/hate relationship with their foam roller. The process of rolling out knots can be quite uncomfortable, but working through the discomfort can help you increase your range of motion and decrease recovery time after a hard workout.

Before you start attacking knots with your foam roller there are three important things to understand:

- When to use a foam roller.
- Basics of using a foam roller.
- Exercises to target specific areas.

The density, texture, size and shape of foam rollers affect how they are used and what they are best for.

Use a Foam Roller

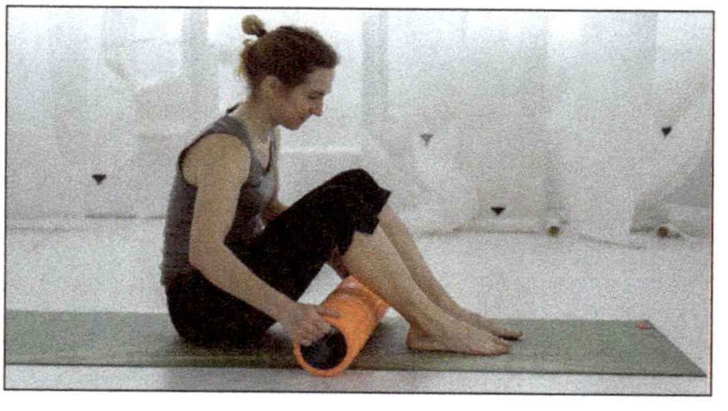

For general muscle soreness, you can use a foam roller just about any time. Some people like to use a roller first thing in the morning or before going to bed. Ana Gonzalez, Certified Personal Trainer and REI employee, suggests that athletes who work out regularly engage in foam rolling immediately before or after a workout for these reasons:

- Before workouts: Rollers may help loosen up muscles, allowing more efficient movement during the workout.
- After workouts: Rollers may help reduce muscle soreness and shorten recovery time.

How to use a Foam Roller

Using a foam roller can be uncomfortable so it's better to be too gentle, rather than too intense, when you're starting out learning how to use a roller. You can adjust your intensity as you learn how your body responds. Generally, you're looking for that "it hurts so good" level of discomfort. Pushing past discomfort into real pain won't speed up results, but it will risk injury. You can actually bruise muscles by rolling too intensely.

Follow these steps to use your foam roller:

- Pinpoint the sore or tight area of your muscle.
- Control your body as you slowly lower the targeted area so it's centered above the roller.
- Lower your body onto the foam roller until you reach a point of discomfort (but not pain) and hold it there.
- Hold for 20–30 seconds.
- The pressure alone provides benefits, but you can also roll slowly back and forth to further stimulate the area.
- Continue to move slowly along the muscle with the roller, stopping and holding in the areas that need more focus.

As you're using your foam roller, experiment with slight adjustments to your body position in order to find the most effective technique. Also, remember to breathe. Many people get so fixated on the sensation of massaging a painful knot that they forget to even take a breath.

Common Foam Roller Exercises

Foam roller exercises are designed to target specific muscle groups.

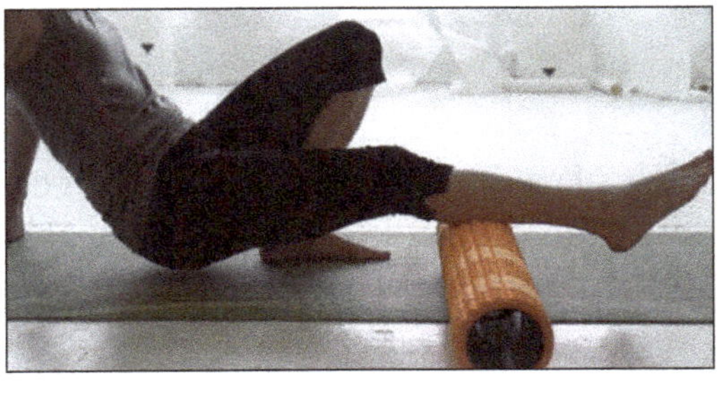

Calf Exercise

While sitting on the ground, extend one leg straight out in front of you and place the foam roller under that calf. Rest your other foot on the floor with the knee bent. Prop yourself up with your arms extended behind you down to the floor. Lift your butt off the floor slightly and begin rolling from your ankle to just below your knee. Roll slowly and when you reach a tender spot, pause and hold the roller for 20–30 seconds before moving on.

You can rotate your leg in and out to work the sides of your calf. Keep your ankle flexed to engage the calf muscle while rolling it. To increase the intensity, place your free foot on top of the shin that is on the roller. This forces your calf to press down harder onto the foam roller.

Repeat on the other leg.

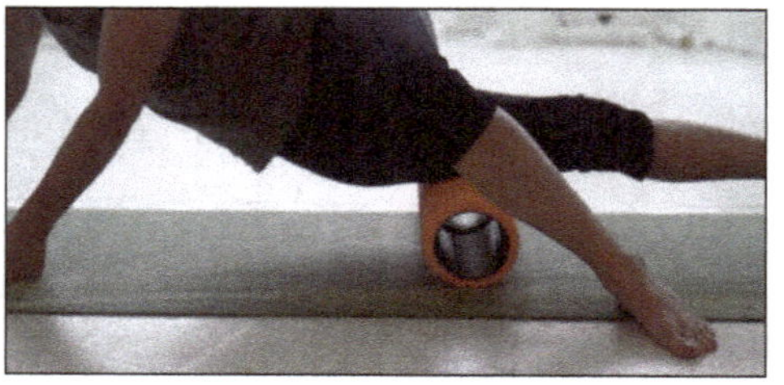

Iliotibial (IT) Band Exercise

Lie down on your side with the roller underneath the side of your quad muscle. Place the foot of your other leg on the floor in front of the leg that's on the roller. Support your upper body with the forearm that's closest to the ground and the hand of your other arm. Roll back and forth along the outer thigh from above your knee to just below the boniest part of your hip, pausing as you go to hold the roller on specific spots for 20–30 seconds. You can lean your body slightly forward or back to adjust the angle of the pressure on your IT band.

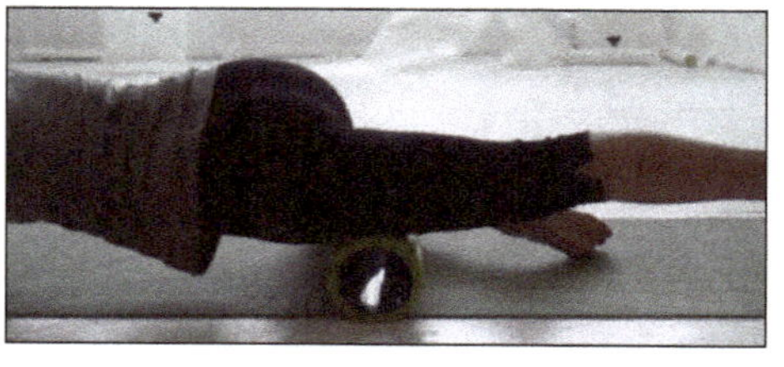

Quadriceps Exercise

Lie face down with the roller placed under your thighs (you can either roll both quads at once or move one leg off to the side and work on one leg at a time.) Prop yourself up on your elbows and roll forward and back from above your knee to your hip.

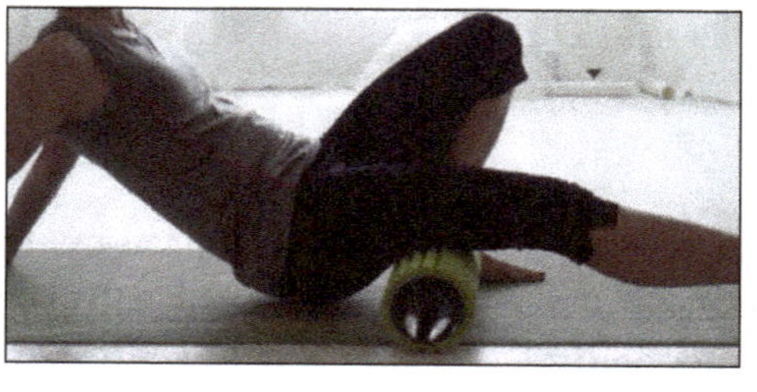

Hamstring Exercise

Sit with the roller positioned under your thighs and your arms extended behind you down to the floor for support. Roll forward and back from above the knee to below your butt. You can roll both hamstrings at once or move one leg off to the side to work one hamstring at a time.

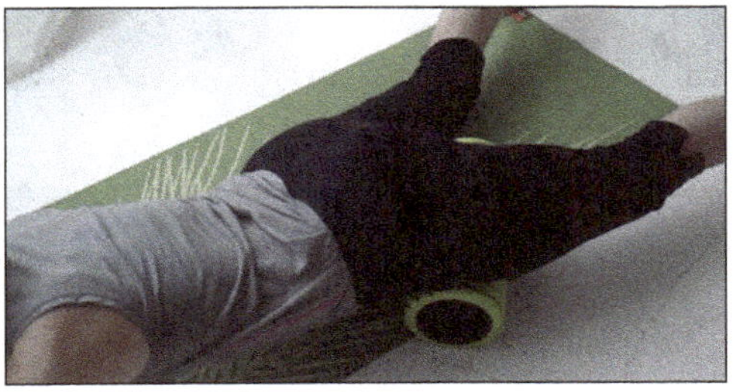

Adductor Exercise

Lie on your stomach and extend one leg out to the side with the knee bent. Place the foam roller near your groin on the side of the extended leg. Prop yourself up on your elbows and roll your inner thigh, from your groin to just above your knee.

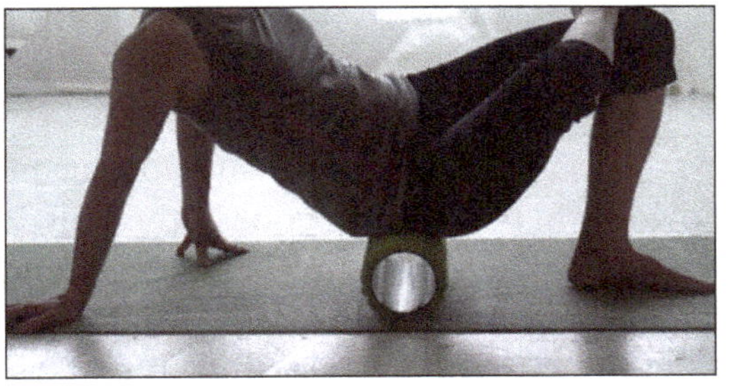

Gluteus Maximus (Glutes) Exercise

To roll your right glute, sit on the foam roller with your knees bent and feet on the floor. Support your upper body with your arms extended down to the ground behind you. Now lift your right foot up and place it on your left knee, creating a position similar to a seated yoga pose. Tilt toward the right and roll forward and back. Repeat on the left side.

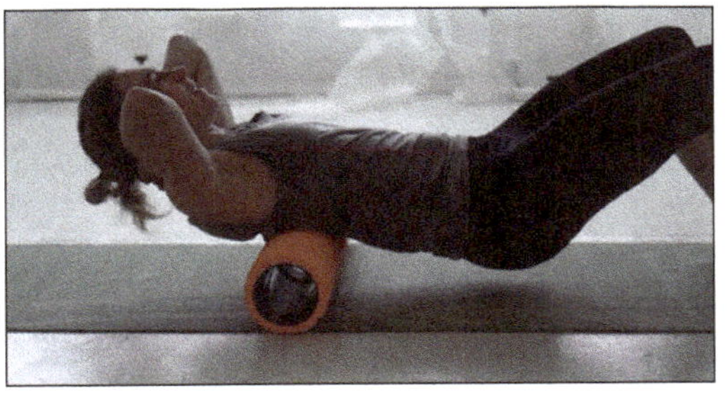

Upper Back Exercise

Lie down on the foam roller with it positioned just below your shoulder blades in the middle of your back and perpendicular to your spine. A foam roller that's about 24–36 in. long is ideal for rolling your back as shorter rollers are not big enough to cover the entire width of your back.

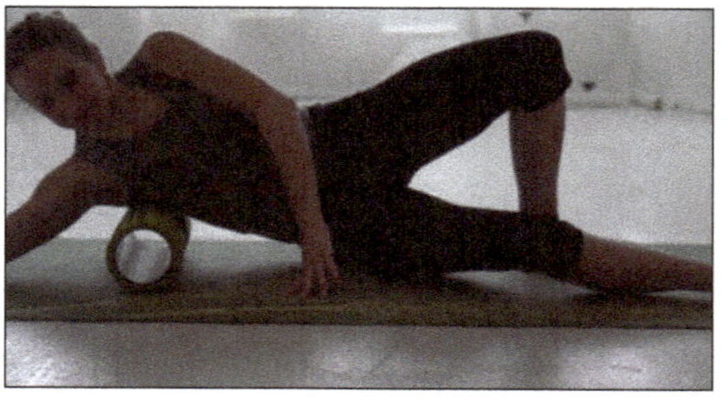

Place your hands behind your neck to support your head but be careful not to pull on your neck. Bring your elbows in and toward your chest to protract your shoulder blades. Bend your knees, lift your butt off the ground and roll forward and back from your mid-back to a few inches below your neck. Be careful around your neck and lower back. These sensitive areas should be avoided.

Latissimi Dorsi (Lats) Exercise

Lie down on one side with the foam roller underneath your armpit and perpendicular to your body. Extend your lower arm in line with your body. You can leave your upper arm and leg stacked on your body, or place them on the floor in front or behind you for support. Roll back and forth from your armpit down to your mid torso. Lean your body forward or backward to get deeper into the muscle. Repeat the exercise on the other side.

Plyometric Exercises

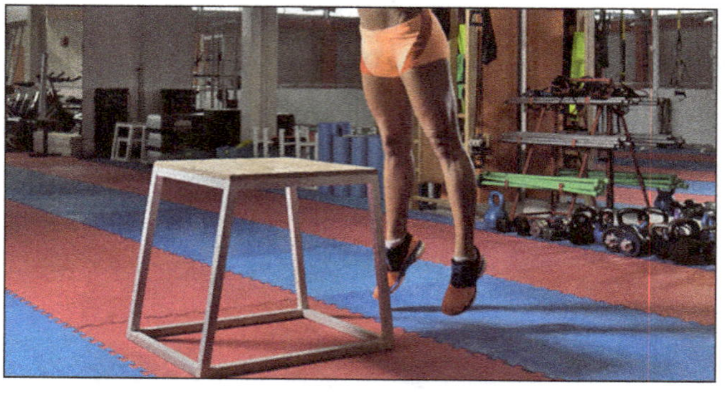

Plyometrics or plyometric exercises are a form of strengthening exercise, incorporating jumping, bounding and hopping movements, which works to increase power in the muscles. Power is used in the vast majority of all sports and so plyometrics can be used to help develop this for most athletes.

- Plyometrics are hopping, jumping and bounding type exercises. They develop stronger, faster muscle contractions.

- A plyometric exercise involves an eccentric muscle contraction, immediately followed by a concentric contraction. This means the muscle contracts, while it is lengthening during the eccentric phase.
- For example, a common plyometric exercise is the depth jump. This involves jumping off a box, landing on both feet in a squatting position, before immediately jumping straight upwards.

Eccentric Contractions

Eccentric contractions produce the maximum amount of force. Therefore, when a muscle contracts eccentrically, the maximum amount of energy is produced. The energy is stored by the elasticity of the muscle. A subsequent concentric contraction must occur as soon as possible to take full advantage of the stored energy in this stretch-shortening cycle.

Types of Plyometric Exercises

- Depth jumps and box drops are popular exercises. To work more on the forward motion, bounding and hoping is best.
- Plyometrics can also be used for improving power in the upper body. These often involve medicine balls ,which when caught require an eccentric contraction to control the motion, followed by a concentric contraction to throw the ball back.
- Push-ups with a clap can also be used. The downward phase of a push-up involves an eccentric contraction of the chest muscles, which is immediately followed by a strong concentric contraction to push back up and clap the hands.

Risks of Plyometric Training

Plyometric training does carry a high injury risk because of its explosive nature. For this reason, athletes should first develop a base level of strength through a standard resistance programme.

Plyometric sessions should be performed a maximum of twice a week and not when you are tired from previous workouts. A thorough warm-up and cool down will also help to prevent injuries, as will a gradual development of the intensity of the exercises performed. Delayed onset muscle soreness is a common complaint.

Functional and Plyometric Exercises

These functional or plyometric type exercises can be performed later in the rehabilitation process. These strengthening exercises are more dynamic and prepare the muscles for when full training is resumed. They include explosive movements such as jumps which work the muscles in a similar way to full training such as sprinting.

Step Back

Step back exercises can be used as late-stage ankle exercises to increase push-off strength, but will also work the hip and bum muscles.

Teaching points:

- Start standing on a small step.
- Take one leg backwards, touch the foot on the floor and push off with the fore-foot to move it back onto the step.
- Alternate legs.
- This can be increased in difficulty by performing on a higher step or at a faster speed.

Muscles Worked:

- Gastrocnemius.
- Soleus.

Resistance band Jumps

The resistance band jump exercise is a great late-stage proprioception test! Hops and jumps can be used in the early stages but using the band adds an extra challenge!

- A resistance band is wrapped around the waist and anchored or held behind the athlete.
- They then perform side to side or forwards and backward jumps.
- The resistance from the band provides a challenge to the balance.

Hopping Exercises

Hopping exercises are important in late-stage rehabilitation in lots of sports. They help to improve balance, proprioception and explosive strength.

- Many variations on hopping exercises are available. Start with a small hop on the spot and gradually increase the height jumped.
- Try hopping to the front, to the side and backwards.
- Try hopping from one leg and landing on the other.
- Equipment such as hoops, agility ladders, and minim hurdles can all be used to add further challenge.

Box Jumps

Box jumps are a form of advanced exercises called plyometrics. They strengthen the entire leg ready for powerful, explosive movements and also aid proprioception development.

Teaching points:

- Numerous exercises can be created using a box or step to jump over.
- To start the athlete may jump sideways over the box, moving rapidly from one foot on one side, to the other foot on the other side. This may also be performed front to back.
- A further progression is high jumps over the box, firstly landing on two feet and progressing to one.

Wrist and Hand Exercises

After a wrist injury, rehabilitation exercises should be performed, but only as soon as pain allows. There is often a balance to be struck between restricting movement of the wrist with splinting or casting to allow it to heal, and the need to restore full range of motion.

These are used to immobilise the wrist allowing the tissues to heal. It is vitally important that any splint or cast is applied arrucately depending on your particular injury.

- Commercially available splints are quick, easy and cheap to fit and are suitable for simple wrist sprains and strains.
- Wrist splints with solid metal stays or 'spoons' restrict movement more and are often used for treatment of Carpal tunnel syndrome.
- Custom made splints and plaster casts are the best option for may injuries if available. Casts are often essential for wrist fractures.

After the Splint/Cast is Removed

- If your wrist has been immobilised for a period of time then it is likely it will be very stiff and weak once the cast or splint is removed.
- Any swelling must be reduced and a compression type wrist support is useful for this.

- You may benefit from wearing a splint overnight, or when returning to sport for protection as you regain full strength and mobility.
- Mobility and stretching exercises are important along with strengthening. Eventually functional or sports specific type exercises should be done before returning to full competition fitness.

Wrist Stretching and Mobility Exercises

Assisted Supinator Stretch

ZThis stretch requires the help of a partner or therapist to stretch the muscles which supinate the wrist (turn the hand over).

- Lie in a relaxed position with the upper arm supported.
- The therapist fully pronates your hand (so the palm faces down).
- A mild stretch may be felt in your wrist and forearm.
- This position can be held for up to a minute, provided it does not cause pain.
- It can also be done with the elbow bent. This reduces the stretch on the biceps muscle to isolate more the supinator.

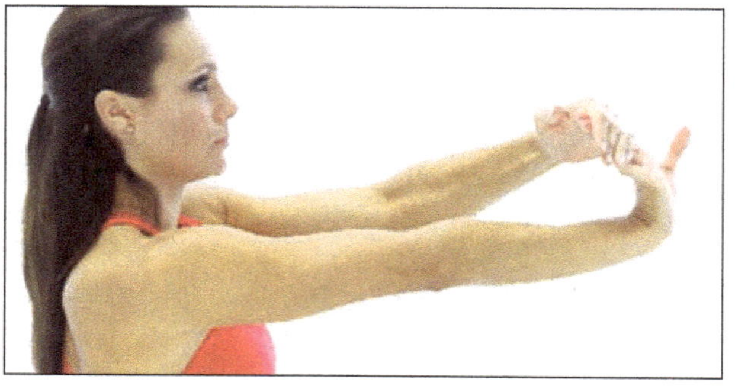

Muscles Stretched:

- Supinator.
- Biceps Brachii.
- Brachioradialis.

Prolonged Wrist Stretches

This exercise aims to increase the range of motion into pronation and supination. Pronation is the movement of turning the hand so the palm faces downwards. Supination is the opposite movements so the palm ends facing upwards.

Muscles Stretched:

In Pronation

- Supinator.
- Biceps Brachii.
- Brachioradialis.

In Supination

- Pronator Teres.
- Pronator Quadratus.

Wrist Strengthening Exercises

Putty Exercises

Putty can be used to strengthen the small muscles of the wrist and hand. This is useful after injuries such as a fracture to any of the small bones in the hand or a wrist, thumb or finger sprain.

- Grip in both hands and pull apart to work on wrist deviation strength.
- It can be held in one hand and twisted with the other to work on wrist extension.
- Putty can also be squeezed to improve grip strength.

Muscles Worked: This depends on the exact exercise, but generally, the intrinsic muscles of the hand are worked to grip it and then the forearm muscles which control wrist extension, flexion, and radial and ulna deviation.

Ulna and Radial Deviation

Ulna and radial deviation are the movements of tilting the wrist from one side to the other. Radial deviation is to move the thumb side of the hand down towards the wrist and ulna deviation is moving the little finger side down.

- To work on ulna deviation, the athlete holds a weighted bar in the hand with the arm by their side so that the palm faces inwards and the weight is at the back, as shown.
- The athlete then tilts the wrist so that the little finger moves upwards.
- To work radial deviation, the arm stays in the same position but the weight is moved to be in front of the hand.
- The wrist is then pulled up so that the thumb moves towards the wrist.

Wrist Strengthening Exercises – Flexion

This wrist flexion exercise can be performed with a dumbbell as shown, or with a resistance band. It is great for strengthening the wrist flexor muscles of the forearm after wrist and elbow injuries.

- To strengthen the muscles which flex the wrist, the athlete sits with the forearm supported and palm facing upwards.
- Starting with the wrist bend downwards and a small weight in the hand, the athlete pulls the wrist upwards, keeping the forearm flat on the table.
- They then slowly reverse this movement.

Muscles worked:

- Flexor Carpi Radialis.
- Flexor Carpi Ulnaris.
- Flexor Digitorum Superficialis.
- Flexor Pollicis Longus.

Wrist Strengthening Exercises – Extension

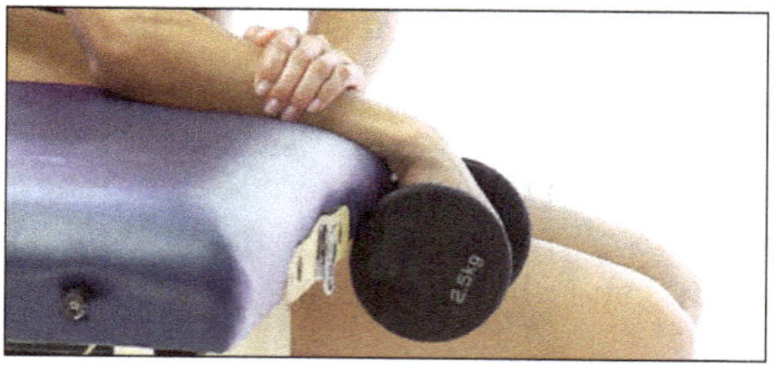

Wrist extension exercises are rarely used in weight training programmes, although it is a great exercise for rehabilitation of injuries such as tennis elbow and sprains/fractures of the wrist.

- Support the arm on a bench or table as shown, with the palm facing downwards.
- Pull the wrist back so that the dumbbell moves towards the body.
- Slowly return to that starting position.

Muscles worked:

- Extensor Carpi Ulnaris,
- Extensor Carpi Radialis Brevis,

- Extensor Carpi Radialis Longus,
- Extensor Pollicis Longus,
- Extensor Digitorum Communis.

Finger Exercises with Rubber Band

Rubberband exercises are a great way for strengthening the finger extensors and is commonly used in treating tennis elbow injuries as the same muscles causing pain at the elbow, also control finger extension.

- A rubber band is placed around the fingers and thumb.
- The athlete spreads the fingers apart as far as possible.
- This can be done on all fingers at once, or between two individual fingers.

Muscles worked:

- Extensor Digitorum Communis.
- Extensor Pollicis Longus.

References

- Stretching-exercises, stretching-exercises: sportsinjuryclinic.net, Retrieved 15 June, 2020
- Foam-roller-exercises, expert-advice: rei.com, Retrieved 21 July, 2020
- Wrist-hand-rehabilitation, rehabilitation-exercises: sportsinjuryclinic.net, Retrieved 21 April, 2020
- Core-strengthening-exercises-that-help-with-back-injury-rehab, education-and-resources-5131: acefitness.org, Retrieved 15 January, 2020
- Wobble-board-exercises: physiotherapy-treatment.com, Retrieved 7 May, 2020
- Sma-lateral-collateral-ligament-sprain-exercises: summitmedicalgroup.com, Retrieved 18 April, 2020
- Pulled-hamstring-exercises, sport-injuries-thigh-pain-back-thigh: sportsinjuryclinic.net, Retrived 14 June, 2020

PERMISSIONS

All chapters in this book are published with permission under the Creative Commons Attribution Share Alike License or equivalent. Every chapter published in this book has been scrutinized by our experts. Their significance has been extensively debated. The topics covered herein carry significant information for a comprehensive understanding. They may even be implemented as practical applications or may be referred to as a beginning point for further studies.

We would like to thank the editorial team for lending their expertise to make the book truly unique. They have played a crucial role in the development of this book. Without their invaluable contributions this book wouldn't have been possible. They have made vital efforts to compile up to date information on the varied aspects of this subject to make this book a valuable addition to the collection of many professionals and students.

This book was conceptualized with the vision of imparting up-to-date and integrated information in this field. To ensure the same, a matchless editorial board was set up. Every individual on the board went through rigorous rounds of assessment to prove their worth. After which they invested a large part of their time researching and compiling the most relevant data for our readers.

The editorial board has been involved in producing this book since its inception. They have spent rigorous hours researching and exploring the diverse topics which have resulted in the successful publishing of this book. They have passed on their knowledge of decades through this book. To expedite this challenging task, the publisher supported the team at every step. A small team of assistant editors was also appointed to further simplify the editing procedure and attain best results for the readers.

Apart from the editorial board, the designing team has also invested a significant amount of their time in understanding the subject and creating the most relevant covers. They scrutinized every image to scout for the most suitable representation of the subject and create an appropriate cover for the book.

The publishing team has been an ardent support to the editorial, designing and production team. Their endless efforts to recruit the best for this project, has resulted in the accomplishment of this book. They are a veteran in the field of academics and their pool of knowledge is as vast as their experience in printing. Their expertise and guidance has proved useful at every step. Their uncompromising quality standards have made this book an exceptional effort. Their encouragement from time to time has been an inspiration for everyone.

The publisher and the editorial board hope that this book will prove to be a valuable piece of knowledge for students, practitioners and scholars across the globe.

INDEX

www.ingramcontent.com/pod-product-compliance
Lightning Source LLC
LaVergne TN
LVHW080622210926
848485LV00003B/197
9781639874286